A Safety Guide on the Use of Essential Oils
(Based on information from worldwide research)

Compiled by

The International School of Aromatherapy

1993

Published by

**Natural by Nature Oils Ltd.
London**

(A Consumer Information Service)

Important Notice:

The nature of toxicity and other hazards is such that it is not realistic to present absolute rules about safety. However, sensible guidelines on the use of essential oils based on reliable information, whenever possible are necessary for their continued safe use. This book is intended only as a general guide on the safety of using essential oils. The information used in this book is based on studies of a random selection of members of the population. The recommendations may not apply to individuals who suffer from idiosyncratic reactions. Medical help should be sought if an adverse reaction occurs or persists.

Copyright © 1993 by The International School of Aromatherapy

All Rights reserved under the provisions of the Copyright Act 1956.

No part of this publication may be reproduced, stored in a retrieval system, or transmitted, in any form, or by any means, electronic, mechanical, photocopying, recording or otherwise; nor be otherwise circulated in any form of binding or cover other than that in which it is published, without the prior written permission of the copyright owner.

ISBN 0 - 9521068 - 0 - 9

Printed and bound in the United Kingdom.

Published by **Natural by Natural Oils Ltd.**
9 Vivian Avenue, Hendon Central, London NW4 3UT, UNITED KINGDOM.

Contents

Foreword

1 Introduction

2 Sources of Information

3 Types of Fragrance Materials

4 Description of Hazards Tested

5 Oral, Dermal & Photo Toxicity (RIFM monographs)

6 Irritation & Sensitisation Reactions (RIFM monographs)

7 Grading of Fragrance Materials including IFRA recommendations

8 Supplement on Fragrance Materials without RIFM monographs

9 Summary and Quick Reference Table on the Essential Oils

10 General Advice on the Use of Essential Oils in Aromathrapy

11 Safety of Aromatherapy in Pregnancy

12 Fragrance Materials Safety Listing

References for the Monographs

Endnote

Foreword

Fragrance materials have been used since antiquity for culinary, therapeutic and perfumery applications. Most of these were obtained from various aromatic plants. With the development of distillation techniques, pure essential oils became available as well as the traditionally crude aromatics like gums, resins and balsams.

In the pursuit of aesthetic refinement, fragrances will always be a part of daily living. The value of essential oils in therapy is also immense and their use in aromatherapy is certainly an important contribution to healthcare. The principal method of administering the essential oils in aromatherapy is by applying them to the skin, where the therapeutic effects are achieved upon absorption. In medical practice, essential oils are also ingested for their therapeutic effects. Consequently safety evaluation of the fragrance materials is necessary to ensure their continued safety in normal use.

Skin contact with the fragrance materials is made on an almost continual basis, especially in the use of cosmetics. This situation may produces the attendant problems of immediate irritation and delayed sensitisation, as well as the possibilities of phototoxic and photoallergic reactions. Beyond the local effects at the site of skin contact, fragrance components can also be absorbed through the skin and exercise systemic effects.

This book has been published as a guide on the safe use of essential oils in the interest of both aromatherapists and the people they treat. The information contained in this book is based on worldwide scientific research by international institutions involved with fragrances. It was originally compiled by the International School of Aromatherapy as part of its educational programme to make reliable safety information available to aromatherapy students, practising aromatherapists, aromatherapy clients, journalists and the general public.

Note: As requested by the publisher, the entries in Chapters 5 and 6 for the RIFM monographs and Chapter 12 for the Safety Listing were re-arranged in alphabetical order to make it easier for readers to find individual entries. In the main part of the book, in Chapters 7, 8 and 9, the entries are retained in their original order.

Chapter 1

Introduction

The potential hazards to human health of using any substance is always of great concern. As modern living involves the availability of all types of substances to the general population, safety guidelines for the use of all categories of substances form an essential part of the regulatory system. The practice of aromatherapy is based on the use of natural fragrance materials, especially plant essential oils. The safety in the use of essential oils, like that of any other substance, involves complex and often confusing factors that require clarification.

Toxicity

The suitability of any drug is assessed according to the balance of its benefits and risks. The greater the benefit, the higher will be the tolerated risk. Absolute safety is unrealistic and impossible to achieve in practice. Every human activity involves risk. The only sensible way to exercise safety is by minimising the risks as much as is practically possible to a generally acceptable level.

The very fact that a substance has medicinal properties makes it potentially toxic if misused. If a drug is so safe as to be completely benign, then it is also devoid of any useful effects and is of little medicinal value. Efficacy cannot exist in the absence of toxicity, and drugs are chosen for their greater effectiveness against their lesser hazards, until comparably effective but less hazardous alternatives are found.

Contra-indications

An important factor in the safe use of drugs is that of contra-indications. Obviously not all drugs are suitable for all conditions. When the use of a particular drug is so unsuitable as to actually worsen the condition it was meant to improve, then it is clearly contra-indicated in that instance. If contra-indications are not observed, then even drugs that do not normally cause adverse reactions may do so.

Dosage

An equally important factor in safety is the quantity of the substance that is administered. Different drugs will produce adverse reactions at different dosages administered to the body. Some very toxic drugs can be used in very small doses in medicine for their beneficial effects; while some of the substances we consume in our food and beverages of very low toxicity can cause serious problems if taken in excess. The very same drug can be both safe and dangerous depending on the amount administered to the body.

Variations

Natural substances obtained from living plants tend to vary in their composition and quality according to numerous ecological and atmospheric factors. Essential oils share this tendency. Government regulatory departments recognise that the toxicity of plants and their constituents are difficult to assess. Many plants including those used as foods have low-level toxicity that is difficult to determine and is generally considered as acceptable. It is only when the level of toxicity is very high that the plant becomes too dangerous for normal use by untrained persons and is prohibited from general availability.

Similarly, the living body is also very complex and intricately connected in structure and function so that reactions to a drug will also vary, sometimes widely, among different individuals. We know for certain that a small percentage of the population will react adversely to any of the essential oils. This situation has to be similarly considered as acceptable. It is not justifiable to prohibit the use of any substance to the rest of the population because of the adverse reactions of the few. It is for those individuals concerned to be aware of their own condition and be judicious in the selection of essential oils as well as other substances, exercising caution in their use.

Those involved in dispensing and administering essential oils may also be prudent by querying the allergic status of potential users. Proper labelling of essential oil containers with adequate safety warnings is also important, and will be very helpful for the uninformed.

Chapter 2

Sources of Information

The most important and extensive assessment of fragrance raw materials in the scientific literature is the series of monographs published by the Research Institute of Fragrance Materials (RIFM) in the 'Food and Cosmetic Toxicology' journal.

In 1966, the RIFM was established as a non-profit making organisation with an independent scientific status, by the principal suppliers of fragrance raw materials from Europe, North America and Japan. The purpose of this Institute was to conduct a systematic investigation of the many aroma chemicals and essential oils used in the perfume industry in order to understand their behaviour. This effort represents an international commitment to ensure the safety of fragrance products as a collective corporate responsibility.

The prime objective of the RIFM is concerned with an assurance of the safety of fragrance raw materials under normal conditions of use. Consequently, the Institute establishes priorities for safety evaluation and testing procedures.

The RIFM maintains its status of scientific independence by confining its investigations to raw materials and does not deal with commercial fragrance products. Scientific information on individual fragrance components is compiled and analysed and where the required data is insufficient, research is conducted by scientific expert panels specialising in toxicology, pharmacology and dermatology to generate further data to supplement the gaps in knowledge. In collating the contributions of investigative work, a reference base of scientific information is now available on the safety of fragrances.

In conducting its work, the RIFM collaborates with several leading national and international organisations. Outstanding among them are:

U.S. Essential Oil Association (EOA)
International Fragrance Association (IFRA)
Cosmetic, Toiletry and Fragrance Association (CTFA)
Flavour and Extract Manufacturers' Association (FEMA)
International Contact Dermatitis Research Group (ICDRG)

The RIFM is purely a test agency and only conducts investigations and publishes its findings. It does not make recommendations. The IFRA, established in 1973, is the advisory agency that makes recommendations on the safe use of fragrance materials. IFRA's recommendations are made, based on the RIFM's test results. The IFRA guidelines and amendments are published periodically in the 'Perfumer and Flavourist' journal.

In the interest of safety, both favourable and unfavourable results of research are published and effectively disseminated, resulting in the removal of hazardous substances from general use. The RIFM programme ensures that the use of fragrances presents minimal risks to the consumer and confirms public expectations in the safety of fragrances.

The resultant data from the RIFM's monographs are intended primarily for the producers in the fragrance industry. However, they have also provided important guidelines for regulatory agencies, health ministries, physicians, dermatologists and consumers worldwide in using fragrance components at safe levels. Equally, they also provide guidelines for the restriction of hazardous fragrance components.

Copies of the RIFM monographs are also sent to the U.S. National Clearing House for Poison Control centres and the Federal U.S. Food and Drug Administration.

The fragrance materials are examined by the RIFM in a ranking order according to the annual amount used in the fragrance industry. Large volume items are examined first, followed by equally important small volume items. By the end of 1992, the RIFM had published over 1000 monographs on fragrance materials of all types. Of these, 196 monographs (about 20%) are on natural fragrance materials of plant origin.

The RIFM is now the largest repository of safety information on fragrance raw materials anywhere in the world. Both RIFM's test results and IFRA's recommendations, when published, are included in this book. Additionally toxicological information from the Registry of Toxic Effects of Chemical Substances, U. S. National Institute of Occupational Safety and Health (NIOSH) is also included for comparison and confirmation.

Chapter 3

Types of Fragrance Materials

Several types of plant fragrance materials are commercially available. All of them are important in perfumery as they offer subtle variations in olfactory qualities. Applications in aromatherapy differ and the values of the different types are not equal. The RIFM have tested fragrance materials of all types. Generally they can be classified into 3 categories depending on their state of purity and the methods used in their extraction.

(I) Essential oils

More accurately known as essences, the pure volatile portion of aromatic plant products normally extracted by distillation are in general usage called essential oils; sometimes they are also called ethereal oils or volatile oils.

The main exceptions to the distillation method of extraction are the citrus essential oils, which are still extracted by physical expression. The citrus fruits are more important for their juices and the fruits are either eaten fresh or their juices are extracted and packaged as drinks. The citrus essential oils are extracted as a by-product of the juice industry. With the increasing importance of the citrus oils in perfumery, a few are now also extracted by distillation.

Essential oils differ from fixed oils which are non-volatile, greasy and stain when they come into contact with paper or clothes. In some species, both essential oils and fixed oils are produced by the same plant and may be extracted separately. Fixed oils are extracted by simple expression, never by distillation. Many of the plant fixed oils are used as salad or cooking oils in food. In aromatherapy, a selection of fixed oils are used as carriers for the essential oils in blends for massage.

This category of essential oils forms the most important group of fragrance materials used in aromatherapy.

(II) Concretes and Absolutes

Concretes and absolutes are also the volatile portions of aromatic plant products, but differ from the pure essential oils by their method of extraction which uses chemical solvents.

Concretes are extracted usually by petroleum ether or benzene and contain waxes so they are usually solid.

Absolutes are further extracted by alcohol to remove the waxes and are purer than concretes.

The solvents are subsequently removed by distilling off in vacuum.

The main disadvantage of concretes and absolutes is the traces of solvent remaining in them, which makes concretes and absolutes more likely to provoke adverse reactions than the distilled essential oils.

The International Fragrance Association (IFRA) issued a guideline in 1989, recommending that the level of benzene as a contaminant in fragrance materials should be kept as low as practicable, not exceeding 10 ppm (parts per million).

(III) Gums, Resins and Balsams

Gums, resins and balsams are crude exudates from plants usually containing some essential oils.

Gums are soluble in water but not in alcohol.

Resins are soluble in alcohol but not in water.

Balsams are mixtures of resins and fixed oils.

More recent advanced technology uses liquid gases (usually carbon dioxide) for extracting the fragrance materials from plants. This method of extraction has the advantage of being suitable for plant parts sensitive to heat without having the problems of trace solvents left in the final extract. The number of essential oils extracted by this method that are commercially available is increasing.

Chapter 4

Description of Hazards tested

The safety information from the RIFM monographs is organised into test results of 5 categories of hazards:

(I). Oral toxicity, (II). Dermal toxicity, (III). Primary Irritation, (IV). Contact Sensitisation & (V). Phototoxicity.

I & II. Oral toxicity & Dermal toxicity

A toxin is a poisonous substance that through its chemical action usually impairs, injures or kills an organism when introduced into its tissues. Toxins are typically capable of inducing antibody formation. Toxicity is the relative degree of a substance being toxic or poisonous.

Oral toxicity is the degree of toxicity of a substance when it is ingested by swallowing. Dermal toxicity is the degree of toxicity of a substance when it is absorbed through the skin. Both types of toxicity are determined by the lethal dose, which is the amount necessary to kill the organism.

Although most drugs tend to be administered orally in medical practice, the number of drugs administered cutaneously is continually increasing. In the use of cosmetics and perfumes and in aromatherapy practice, dermal application is more important. Consequently dermal toxicity will be more significant for this study.

III. Irritation reaction

Irritation is a reaction to a substance by an organism resulting in inflammation and soreness when the substance is brought into contact with it. Substances that produce such a reaction are considered to be irritants. Dermal irritation is the reaction to an irritant substance when the substance is brought into contact with the skin. This is a localised type of reaction and does not involve a systemic response.

Additional notes on irritation -

The recommendations for the safe use of fragrance materials by the IFRA are generally applicable worldwide. However some variations among population groups do occur and recent research by Japanese universities have shown that Oriental (Chinese, Japanese, Korean) skins tend to be more sensitive to irritant substances than the skins of people from Europe or North America. The regulating agencies in Japan therefore have their own codes for the safe use of fragrance materials. These codes extend rather than replace the IFRA guidelines.
[Dragoco Report 7th May 1982]

Other factors also affect skin sensitivity to irritation. A Japanese study by the Departments of Dermatology of Toho University Medical School and Kansai Medical School in 1979 involving approximately 200 human volunteers over an 8 year period using 270,000 close patch tests have shown the following factors to affect skin sensitivity to irritation -

1. Change of season (known to trigger illness in certain people).
More sensitivity among the test volunteers occurred in October when the season was changing from summer to autumn and in March when the season was changing from winter to spring. (No tests were conducted in summer due to the excessive amount of perspiration produced which affected the testing).

2. Sex.
Men are 2.5 times more sensitive than women.

3. Illness and stress-related situations.
(marriage, pregnancy, divorce, bereavement)
Individuals experienced an increase in skin sensitivity when suffering from stress or illness; the same individuals were less sensitive when not ill or less stressed.

There seemed to be no relation between chemical structure and skin reaction.
[Study of skin irritation caused by perfume materials (1979) Perfumer & Flavourist Vol.4 No.4]

Materials which produced adverse reactions in more than 1% of the test volunteers were excluded from normal use.

IV. Sensitisation reaction

Sensitisation is an allergic reaction to a substance by an organism that involves the interaction of its immune system with the substance. Substances that are capable of inducing an immune response from an organism are considered to be antigens. The antigens interact with the lymphocytes (lymph cells) causing the formation of antibodies that react with and render the antigens harmless. When an antigen induces an immune response at the first exposure, the organism will experience an altered bodily reactivity to subsequent exposure to the same or similar antigens, causing exaggerated reactions (like sneezing and itching). This is the allergic condition. Contact sensitisation is the allergic reaction to an antigen substance when the substance is brought into contact with the skin. [Perfumer & Flavourist (1976) Vol.1 No.2 pgs.32-4]

More recent findings on sensitisation -

Sensitisation is a response of the immune system but it is not an antigen-antibody reaction. Skin sensitisation is a delayed type humoral immune response mediated by the T-cells. The incomplete allergen bonds with a protein in the skin. Cells in the stratum germinativum of the skin interact with this allergen, migrate to the thymus gland and prime the other uninitiated thymus T-cells. When the sensitised T-cells leaving the thymus gland come into contact with the allergen, they liberate lymphokines, attracting other leukocytes to the area and raise the temperature in an attempt to rid the material producing the inflammation .
[Hazardous Substances - Supplementary Definition of Strong Sensitizers (Aug.14th 1986) U.S. Federal Regulation 51(157):29094]

V. Phototoxic reaction

Certain substances react chemically with an organism only in the presence of radiation. These substances are considered to be phototoxic. A phototoxic reaction is the response of an organism to a substance rendering the skin susceptible to damage such as blisters or sunburn and subsequent hyper-pigmentation, upon exposure to light, especially ultra-violet light. Such substances are considered to be phototoxic. The phototoxic reaction only occurs on the skin areas that are exposed to either natural or simulated sunlight.

Photoallergic reactions

A photoallergenic reaction is the response of an organism to a substance causing allergic sensitivity to light. Some fragrance materials possess phototoxic properties but as a group, they generally tend not to be photoallergenic. They are therefore not tested for this hazard.

Some substances are also capable of inducing carcinogenic, mutagenic and teratogenic effects on organisms.

Carcinogenesis

Carcinogenesis is the action of a carcinogen, which is a substance or agent that can produce cancer. A cancer is a malignant tumour of potentially unlimited growth that expands locally by invasion and systemically by developing similar lesions in the new location.

Mutagenesis

Mutagenesis is the action of a mutagen, which is a substance or agent that can produce genetic mutation. Mutation is the relatively permanent physical or biochemical change in a developing embryo resulting in deformity.

Teratogenesis

Teratogenesis is the action of a teratogen, which is a substance or agent that can produce developmental malformation in a foetus resulting in monstrous growths.

A few carcinogenic tests are conducted for selected fragrance materials, but there is no evidence that fragrance material poses any potential hazards of mutagenicity or teratogenicity. Tests are therefore not conducted for these hazards.

Chapter 5

Oral, Dermal and Photo-toxicity of Natural Fragrance Materials

Except for the occasional reports of accidental human poisoning, all systematic toxicity studies are performed on animals. Unfortunately, there are at present no alternative methods to animal testing for determining toxicity values without endangering human health. In 1981, US$1 million was made available in America to investigate alternatives to animal testing. [Dragoco Report 7th May 1982]

One promising alternative is the use of microbes and cell culture, but the technology is not advanced enough yet to be practically useful.

Animals like humans vary in their reactions to a particular substance. Consequently, toxicity values are determined as an average threshold limit. The usual method is the LD50 which is the lethal dose of 50% of the number of tested animals. The group of test animals is administered increasing amounts of the test substance until half the number of animals die. The amount administered at this point is then taken as the lethal dose of that substance.

Rats are generally used for testing oral toxicity and rabbits for dermal toxicity; occasionally mice are used instead of rats and guineapigs instead of rabbits. Values listed in the tables for oral and dermal toxicity apply to rats and rabbits respectively, unless otherwise indicated. Occasionally other species of animals are also involved in the tests.

Testings with fragrance materials of very low toxicity are stopped at 5g/kg and when no test animals die at this concentration, the toxicity value is simply considered to be greater than 5g/kg without determining the actual toxic dose. Subsequently the test animals are not subjected to further increase of the test dosage.

Acute oral and dermal toxicity is determined only as a general measure of toxicity. Additional toxicological data is limited to the use of fragrance materials as perfumes on the skin, as distinct from use as flavourings in foods and drinks.

Rats are considered to be the most suitable animals for testing oral toxicity and the results are supposed to closely reflect the toxic effects on humans. However, some plants toxic to humans are not toxic to rats and conversely some plants which are toxic to rats are not toxic to humans. Dermal toxicity involves absorption of the substances through the skin. The rate of dermal absorption also differs between rabbit skin and human skin; rabbit skin apparently being more absorptive.

Testing for phototoxic reaction is also conducted when it is considered to be pertinent. 0.2ml of the fragrance material at 100% is applied on 5 cubic cm of the skins of hairless mice and miniature swine, followed by UVA irradiation from fluorescent backlight (PUVA phototherapy lamps) or xenon arc solar simulator lamps for 1 hour. The skins are subsequently examined for indications of phototoxic reactions.

The listed fragrance materials have been tested and shown to be non-phototoxic unless otherwise stated.

Results from animal testing cannot be considered to apply to humans precisely, as animal and human physiology differs quite significantly in many ways. Equally, the physiology between animal species also differs. The results from these tests only provide a rough guide to toxic levels of the tested substances. Toxicity data should therefore be interpreted with this consideration.

The information included in this chapter is the most reliable so far available and is presented here, with reservations, until information that is more reliable and is obtained by more humane methods becomes available.

NATURAL FRAGRANCE MATERIALS	oral toxicity (rats)	dermal toxicity (rabbits)
001 ale oil (Pinus sp.)	>5g/kg	>5g/kg
002 almond oil, bitter (Prunus amygdalus)	0.96g/kg	1.2g/kg

Human ingestion of 7.5ml has resulted in death. High toxicity due to hydrocyanic acid (also called 'prussic acid').

003 almond oil, bitter (Prunus amygdalus) [FFPA]	1.5ml/kg	>3ml/kg
004 ambrette seed oil (Hibiscus abelmoschus)	>5g/kg	>5g/kg
005 amyris oil (Amyris balsamifera) [acetylated]	>5g/kg	>5g/kg
006 angelica root oil (Angelica archangelica)	11.16g/kg 2.2g/kg (mice)	>5g/kg

Tolerated dose in rats at daily intake for 8 weeks was 1.5g/kg but even at 0.5-1.0g/kg daily dose caused decrease in weight and activity among the tested animals. Lethal oral dose in rats is 11.16g/kg when death is preceded by severe liver and kidney damage but test animals surviving for 3 days recovered completely from any liver or kidney damage.

Exposure to simulated sunlight for 1 hr. produced -
positive phototoxic reactions from 3%; slight reaction at 1.5%; not phototoxic at 0.78%

007 angelica seed oil (Angelica archangelica)	>5g/kg	>5g/kg
008 anise oil (Pimpinella anisum)	2.25g/kg	>5g/kg

not tested for phototoxicity

009 armoise oil (Artemisia vulgaris)	0.37g/kg (mice)	>5g/kg (guineapigs)
010 basil oil, sweet (Ocimum basilicum)	1.4g/kg	>5g/kg
011 bay oil (Pimenta racemosa)	1.8g/kg	>5ml/kg

not tested for phototoxicity

NATURAL FRAGRANCE MATERIALS	oral toxicity (rats)	dermal toxicity (rabbits)
012 benzoin resinoid (Styrax benzoin)	10g/kg	8.9g/kg

not tested for phototoxicity

013 bergamot oil, expressed (Citrus bergamia)	>10g/kg	>20g/kg

Severe phototoxic reactions have been reported in humans after exposure to natural and simulated sunlight. Also reported to be phototoxic to mice and swine. Photodermatitis caused by expressed bergamot oil is attributed to the non-volatile content of bergapten occurring at up to 0.4%. The phototoxic reaction is neutralised by reducing the bergapten content to 0.001% and below.

014 bergamot oil, rectified (Citrus bergamia)	>10g/kg	>20g/kg

[rectification under vacuum completely removes all non-volatile residues including the furocoumarins that are present in the expressed oil and renders the essential oil non-phototoxic: FCF - furocoumarin free]

015 birch tar oil (Betula pendula)	>5g/kg	>2g/kg
016 sweet birch oil (Betula lenta)	1.7g/kg	>5g/kg
017 bois de rose oil (Aniba rosaeodora)	4.3g/kg	>5g/kg
018 bois de rose oil (Aniba rosaeodara) [acetylated]	>5g/kg	>5g/kg
019 boldo leaf oil (Peumus boldus)	0.13g/kg	0.9g/kg

An oral dose of 0.07g/kg produced convulsions in rats, with death occurring at 0.13g/kg.

020 Brazilian sassafras oil (Ocotea cymbarum)	1.58g/kg	>5g/kg
021 cabreuva oil (Murocarpus frondosus & fastigiatus)	>5g/kg	>5g/kg
022 cade tar oil, rectified (Juniperus oxycedrus)	8.0g/kg	>5g/kg

Oral toxicity signs in rats included depression and gastrointestinal irritation.

NATURAL FRAGRANCE MATERIALS	oral toxicity (rats)	dermal toxicity (rabbits)
023 cajeput oil (Melaleuca leucodendron)	3.87g/kg	>5g/kg
024 calamus oil (Acorus calamus)	0.8-8.8g/kg	>5g/kg (guineapigs)

Oral toxic signs in rats include convulsions and severe liver and kidney damage, but test animals surviving for 3 days recovered completely from any liver or kidney damage. Daily oral doses at 0.25-2.0% of food intake for 18 weeks caused liver and heart changes, the latter with slight myocardial degeneration characterised by muscle fibrosis and necrosis.

Carcinogenesis in rats:
fed to rats at 0.05-0.5% in the diet, calamus oil caused malignant tumours to develop in the intestines after 59 weeks.

025 camphor oil, white (Cinnamomum camphora)	5.1ml/kg	>5ml/kg

not tested for phototoxicity

026 camphor oil, yellow (Cinnamomum camphora)	3.3-4.15g/kg	>5g/kg
027 camphor oil, brown (Cinnamomum camphora)	2.53ml/kg	>4ml/kg
028 cananga oil (Cananga odorata)	>5g/kg	>5g/kg

not tested for phototoxicity

029 caraway oil (Carum carvi)	3.5ml/kg	1.78ml/kg

Reported low-level phototoxic reaction at 100% not considered to be significant.

030 cardamom oil (Elettaria cardamomum)	>5g/kg	>5g/kg
031 carrot seed oil (Daucus carota)	>5g/kg (mice)	>5g/kg (guineapigs)
032 cascarilla oil (Croton eluteria)	>5g/kg (mice)	>5g/kg

NATURAL FRAGRANCE MATERIALS	oral toxicity (rats)	dermal toxicity (rabbits)
033 cassia oil (Cinnamomum cassia)	2.8ml/kg	0.32ml/kg

Reported low-level phototoxic reaction at 100% not considered to be significant.

034 cedarwood oil, Atlas (Cedrus atlantica)	>5g/kg	>5g/kg
035 celery seed oil (Apium graveolens)	>5g/kg	>5g/kg

Workers harvesting and preparing celery for canning have been reported to suffer from phototoxic reactions producing blisters and lesions. The dermatitis was confined to the upper limbs and associated with itching, apparently caused by contact with the plant oil.

036 chamomile oil, German (Matricaria chamomilla)	>5g/kg	>5g/kg
037 chamomile oil, Roman (Anthemis nobilis)	>5g/kg	>5g/kg
038 chenopodium oil (Chenopodium ambrosioides)	0.255g/kg 0.38ml/kg (mice) 0.3-0.6ml/kg (chicken) 0.28-0.4ml/kg (dogs)	0.415g/kg

Several cases of fatal human poisoning have been reported. Toxic effects include skin and mucous-membrane irritation, headache, vertigo, nausea, vomiting, constipation, tinnitus, temporary deafness, diplopia (double vision) and blindness, transient stimulation followed by depression of the central nervous system leading to delirium and coma, occasional convulsions, circulatory collapse due to vasomotor paralysis and sometimes pulmonary oedema. Chenopodium oil is also toxic to the kidneys and liver.

039 cinnamon bark oil (Cinnamomum zeylanicum)	3.4ml/kg	0.69ml/kg

Reported low-level phototoxicity reaction at 100% not considered to be significant.

040 cinnamon leaf oil (Cinnamomum zeylanicum)	2.65g/kg	>5g/kg
041 citronella oil (Cymbopogon nardus)	>5g/kg	4.7ml/kg

not tested for phototoxicity

NATURAL FRAGRANCE MATERIALS	oral toxicity (rats)	dermal toxicity (rabbits)
042 clove bud oil (Eugenia caryophyllata)	2.65-3.72g/kg*	5g/kg

Daily oral doses in rats at 0.35-0.7g/kg for 8 weeks were well tolerated; higher doses cause inactivity and weight loss.

043 clove leaf oil (Eugenia caryophyllata)	1.37g/kg	1.2g/kg
044 clove stem oil (Eugenia caryophyllata)	2.0-3.72g/kg*	>5g/kg

Daily oral doses in rats at 0.35-0.7g/kg for 8 weeks were well tolerated; higher doses cause inactivity and weight loss.

045 cognac oil, green (Vitis vinifera)	>5g/kg	>5g/kg (guineapigs)
046 copaiba balsam (Copaifera reticulata)	5g/kg	>5g/kg
047 copaiba oil (Copaifera reticulata)	>5g/kg	>5g/kg

not tested for phototoxicity

048 coriander oil (Coriandrum sativum)	4.13g/kg	>5g/kg

not tested for phototoxicity

049 cornmint oil (Mentha arvensis)	1.24g/kg	>5g/kg
050 costus root absolute & concrete (Saussurea lappa)	3.4g/kg	>5g/kg
051 costus root oil (Saussurea lappa)	3.4g/kg	>5g/kg
052 cubeb oil (Piper cubeba)	>5g/kg	>5g/kg
053 cumin oil (Cuminum cyminum)	2.5ml/kg	3.56ml/kg

Reported to have distinct phototoxic reactions at 100%.

NATURAL FRAGRANCE MATERIALS	oral toxicity (rats)	dermal toxicity (rabbits)
054 cypress oil (Cupressus sempervirens)	>5g/kg	>5g/kg
055 davana oil (Artemisia pallens)	>5g/kg	>5g/kg
056 deertongue absolute (Liatris odoratissima)	>5g/kg	>5g/kg
057 deertongue incolore (Liatris odoratissima)	0.73g/kg	3.67g/kg
058 dill herb oil (Anethum graveolens) The plant has been reported to be a photosensitising agent.	4.0ml/kg	>5g/kg
059 dill seed oil, Indian (Anethum sowa)	4.6g/kg	>5g/kg
060 Douglas fir balsam (Pseudotsuga taxifolia)	>5g/kg	>5g/kg
061 eau de brouts absolute (Citrus aurantium)	>5g/kg	>5g/kg
062 elecampane/alantroot oil (Inula helenium) *not tested for phototoxicity*	not tested	not tested
063 elemi oil (Canarium commune)	3-3.8g/kg >5g/kg (mice)	5g/kg
064 (Eucalyptus globulus) oil (*) - The RIFM did not test for oral toxicity. This value was provided by the National Institute of Occupational Safety and Health (NIOSH) of the United States. Oral toxicity for the main constituent of eucalyptus oil, eucalyptol was determined by the RIFM as 2.48g/kg.	4.44g/kg (*)	>5g/kg
065 (Eucalyptus citriodora) oil	>5g/kg	2.48g/kg

NATURAL FRAGRANCE MATERIALS	oral toxicity (rats)	dermal toxicity (rabbits)
066 (Eucalyptus citriodora) oil [acetylated]	9.5ml/kg	>5g/kg
067 fennel seed oil, bitter (Foeniculum vulgare)	4.52g/kg	>5g/kg
068 fennel seed oil, sweet (Foeniculum vulgare)	3.8g/kg	>5g/kg
069 fenugreek absolute (Trigonella foenum-graecum)	>5g/kg	>2g/kg
070 fig leaf absolute (Ficus carica)	not tested	not tested

Reported to be strongly phototoxic at 12.5%; tested even at 0.001% still produced phototoxic reactions in half the test animals.

071 fir cone oil, silver (Abies alba)	>5g/kg	>5g/kg
072 fir needle oil, silver (Abies alba)	>5g/kg	>5g/kg
073 fir balsam, Canadian (Abies balsamea) *not tested for phototoxicity*	>5g/kg	>5g/kg
074 fir needle oil, Canadian (Abies balsamea)	>5g/kg	>5g/kg
075 fir needle oil, Siberian (Abies sibirica) *not tested for phototoxicity*	10.2g/kg	>3g/kg
076 flouve oil (Anthoxanthum odoratum)	3.7-4.5g/kg	5g/kg
077 foin absolute (Anthoxanthum odoratum)	>5g/kg	>5g/kg

NATURAL FRAGRANCE MATERIALS	oral toxicity (rats)	dermal toxicity (rabbits)
078 galbanum oil (Ferula galbaniflua) *not tested for phototoxicity*	>5g/kg	>5g/kg
079 galbanum resin (Ferula galbaniflua)	>5g/kg	>5g/kg
080 genet absolute (Spartium junceum)	>5g/kg	>5g/kg
081 geranium oil, Algerian (Pelargonium graveolens)	not tested	>5g/kg (guineapigs)
082 geranium oil, Bourbon (Pelargonium graveolens)	>5g/kg	2.5g/kg
083 geranium oil, Moroccan (Pelargonium graveolens)	not tested	>5g/kg (guineapigs)
084 ginger oil (Zingiber officinale) **Reported low-level phototoxic reactions at 100% not considered to be significant.**	>5g/kg	>5g/kg
085 grapefruit oil, expressed (Citrus paradisi)	>5g/kg	>5g/kg
086 guaiacwood oil (Bulnesia sarmienti)	>5g/kg	>5g/kg
087 gurjun balsam (Dipterocarpus turbinatus & tuberculatus)	>5g/kg	>5g/kg
088 gurjun oil (Dipterocarpus turbinatus & tuberculatus)	>5g/kg	>5g/kg
089 hibawood oil (Thujopsis dolabrata)	>5g/kg	>5g/kg
090 ho leaf oil (Cinnamomum camphora) *not tested for phototoxicity*	3.27g/kg	>5g/kg

NATURAL FRAGRANCE MATERIALS	oral toxicity (rats)	dermal toxicity (rabbits)
091 honeysuckle absolute (Lonicera caprifolium)	not tested	not tested

Reported to produce minimal phototoxic reactions at 100%; not phototoxic below 50% in benzene or below 70% in methanol.

092 hyacinth absolute (Hyacinthus orientalis)	4.2g/kg	>1.25g/kg
093 hyssop oil (Hyssopus officinalis)	1.4ml/kg	5ml/kg
094 immortelle absolute (Helichrysum angustifolium)	4.4g/kg	>5g/kg
095 immortelle oil (Helichrysum angustifolium)	>5g/kg	>5g/kg
096 jasmine absolute (Jasminum officinale)	>5g/kg	>5g/kg
097 jonquil absolute (Narcissus jonquilla)	not tested	not tested
098 juniper berry oil (Juniperus communis)	8.0g/kg	>5g/kg
099 juniper oil, Phoenician (Juniperus phoenicia)	>5g/kg	>5g/kg
100 karo karounde absolute (Leptactina senegambica)	1.4g/kg (mice)	>5g/kg (guineapigs)
101 labdanum/cyste absolute (Cistus ladaniferus)	>5g/kg	>5g/kg
102 labdanum/cyste oil (Cistus ladaniferus)	8.98g/kg	>5g/kg

not tested for phototoxicity

103 laurel leaf oil (Laurus nobilis)	3.95g/kg	>5g/kg

NATURAL FRAGRANCE MATERIALS	oral toxicity (rats)	dermal toxicity (rabbits)
104 lavandin absolute (Lavandula hybrida)	>5g/kg (mice)	>5g/kg >5g/kg(guineapigs)
105 lavandin oil (Lavandula hybrida)	>5g/kg	>5g/kg
106 lavandin oil (Lavandula hybrida) [acetylated]	>5g/kg	>5g/kg
107 lavender absolute (Lavandula officinalis) *not tested for phototoxicity*	4.25g/kg	>5g/kg(guineapigs)
108 lavender oil (Lavandula officinalis)	>5g/kg	>5g/kg
109 lavender oil, spike/aspic (Lavandula latifolia) *not tested for phtotoxicity*	3.8g/kg	>2g/kg
110 lemon oil, distilled (Citrus limon)	>5g/kg	>5g/kg
111 lemon oil, expressed (Citrus limon) **Reported low-level to distinct phototoxic reactions at 100%.**	>5g/kg	>5g/kg
112 lemongrass oil, E. Indian (Cymbopogon citratus)	5.6g/kg	>2g/kg
113 lemongrass oil, W. Indian (Cymbopogon citratus)	>5g/kg	>5g/kg
114 lemonmint oil (Mentha citrata)	>5g/kg	>5g/kg(guineapigs)
115 lime oil, distilled (Citrus aurantifolia)	>5g/kg	>5g/kg

NATURAL FRAGRANCE MATERIALS	oral toxicity (rats)	dermal toxicity (rabbits)
116 lime oil, expressed (Citrus aurantifolia)	not tested	not tested

Reported to be phototoxic at 100% in humans, mice and swine. A case of photodermatitis has been reported.

117 linaloe wood oil (Bursera delpechiana)	>5g/kg	>5g/kg
118 litsea oil (Litsea cubeba)	>5g/kg	4.8g/kg
119 lovage oil (Levisticum officinale)	3.4g/kg (mice)	>5g/kg (guineapigs)
120 mace oil (Myristica fragans)	3.64g/kg	>5g/kg
121 mandarin oil, expressed (Citrus reticulata)	>5g/kg	>5g/kg
122 marjoram oil (Origanum marjorana)	2.24g/kg	>5g/kg

not tested for phototoxicity

123 mastic absolute (Pisticia lentiscus)	>5g/kg	>5g/kg
124 mimosa absolute (Acacia decurrens)	>5g/kg	>5g/kg (guineapigs)
125 myrrh absolute (Commiphora myrrha)	not tested	not tested
126 myrrh oil (Commiphora myrrha)	1.65g/kg	not tested
127 myrtle oil (Myrtus communis)	7.36g/kg 4.46g/kg (mice)	>5g/kg (guineapigs)

Daily oral doses in rats at higher than 1.5ml/kg for 3 weeks caused an initial weight loss, regained after a few days; doses of 2.7ml/kg caused a loss of righting reflexes. By an adaptive mechanism, the rats developed a tolerance to higher doses; after a daily dose of 2ml/kg for 2 weeks, the mean lethal dose in the surviving rats increased to 6.6ml/kg. At the lethal dose of 7.36ml/kg death was attributable to central nervous system depression.

NATURAL FRAGRANCE MATERIALS	oral toxicity (rats)	dermal toxicity (rabbits)
128 narcissus absolute (Narcissus poetieus)	>5g/kg (mice)	>5g/kg (guineapigs)
129 neroli/orange flower absolute (Citrus aurantium)	>5g/kg	>5g/kg

not tested for phtotoxicity

130 neroli/orange flower oil (Citrus aurantium)	4.4-4.6g/kg	>5g/kg
131 nutmeg oil (Myristica fragans)	0.64-2.6g/kg 5-6g/kg (mice) 5.8-6.2g/kg (hamsters)	>10ml/kg

In animals, lethal doses cause fatty degeneration of the liver and central nervous system paralysis. The liver changes have been attributed to the myristicin content of nutmeg oil.

Several cases of human intoxication have been reported.
In 1960, 2 Swedish girls ingesting 15-25g of powdered nutmeg experienced impaired visual perception, sleeping continuously for 40 hours and waking up in an euphoric state; the intoxication is dose dependent and their symptoms lasted for 10 days.

not tested for phototoxicity

132 oakmoss concrete (Evernia prunastri)	2.9g/kg	>5g/kg
133 olibanum absolute (Boswellia carterii)	not tested	not tested
134 olibanum gum (Boswellia carterii)	>5g/kg	>5g/kg

not tested for phototoxicity

135 bitter orange oil, expressed (Citrus aurantium)	>5g/kg	>10g/kg

Reported distinct phototoxic reactions at 100%.
Sensitisation of the skin to light following the use of cologne containing oil of bitter orange has been reported in some individuals.

136 sweet orange oil, expressed (Citrus sinensis)	>5g/kg	>5g/kg

NATURAL FRAGRANCE MATERIALS	oral toxicity (rats)	dermal toxicity (rabbits)
137 oregano oil (Origanum vulgare)	1.85g/kg	0.48g/kg
138 orris absolute (Iris pallida)	9.4g/kg	not tested
139 palmarosa oil (Cymbopogon martini)	>5g/kg	>5g/kg
140 parsley herb oil (Petroselinum sativum)	3.3g/kg	>5g/kg
141 parsley seed oil (Petroselinum sativum)	3.96g/kg 1.52g/kg (mice)	>5g/kg (guineapigs)

The plant is toxic to chickens; a dose of 17.8g/kg caused diarrhoea, convulsions, paralysis and death.
A single dose of 10ml/kg of parsley seed extract in mice caused anuria, drowsiness, dyspnoea and hyperaemia of the viscera with death after 24-60 hours. No toxic effects were observed in dogs at doses as high as 60g/kg.

142 patchouli oil (Pogostemon cablin)	>5g/kg	>5g/kg
143 pennyroyal oil (Mentha pulegium)	0.4g/kg	4.2g/kg
144 pepper oil, black (Piper nigrum)	>5g/kg	>5g/kg

Reported low-level phototoxic reaction at 100% not considered to be significant.

145 perilla oil (Perilla frutescens)	>5g/kg 2.77g/kg (mice)	>5g/kg
146 Peru balsam (Myroxylon pereirae)	>5g/kg	>10g/kg
147 Peru balsam oil (Myroxylon pereirae)	2.36-3.5ml/kg	2 - 5g/kg

NATURAL FRAGRANCE MATERIALS	oral toxicity (rats)	dermal toxicity (rabbits)
148 Peruvian mastic oil (Schinus molle)	>5g/kg	>5g/kg
149 petitgrain oil, Bigarade (Citrus aurantium)	>5g/kg	>2g/kg
150 petitgrain oil, Paraguay (Citrus aurantium)	>5g/kg	>5g/kg
151 petitgrain oil, lemon (Citrus limon)	>5g/kg	>5g/kg
152 pimento berry oil (Pimenta officinalis)	not tested	not tested
153 pimento leaf oil (Pimenta officinalis)	3.6ml/kg	2.82ml/kg
154 pine oil, pumilo (Pinus pumilo)	10.64g/kg	>5g/kg
155 pine oil, yarmor (Pinus palustris)	3.2g/kg	5g/kg
156 pine oil, Scots (Pinus sylvestris)	6.88g/kg	>5g/kg
157 rose absolute, French (Rosa centifolia)	>5g/kg	uncertain
158 rose oil, Bulgarian (Rosa damascena)	>5g/kg	2.5g/kg
159 rose oil, Moroccan (Rosa centifolia)	>5g/kg	>2.5g/kg
160 rose oil, Turkish (Rosa damascena)	>5g/kg	>2.5g/kg

NATURAL FRAGRANCE MATERIALS	oral toxicity (rats)	dermal toxicity (rabbits)
161 rosemary oil (Rosmarinus officinalis)	5g/kg	>10ml/kg

not tested for phototoxicity

162 rue oil (Ruta graveolens)	>5g/kg leaves-2.54g/kg (mice) fruits-3.73g/kg (mice)	>5g/kg

Large oral doses in rabbits and guineapigs causes dyspnoea, diarrhoea, torpor and sometimes haematemesis and weight loss.

Taken internally, rue oil may produce haemorrhages. Ingestion of large quantities of rue oil causes epigastric pain, nausea, vomiting, confusion, convulsions and death. Abortion may also result.
Exposure to simulated sunlight for 1 hr produced -
distinct phototoxic reactions from 3%; slight reaction at 1.5%; negative results at 0.78%

163 sage oil, clary French (Salvia sclarea)	5.6g/kg	>2g/kg
164 sage oil, clary Russian (Salvia sclarea)	not tested	not tested
165 sage oil, Dalmatian (Salvia officinalis)	2.6g/kg	>5g/kg

not tested for phototoxicity

166 sage oil, Spanish (Salvia lavandulaefolia)	>5g/kg	>5g/kg
167 sandalwood oil (Santalum album)	5.58g/kg	>5g/kg
168 sassafras oil (Sassafras albidum)	1.9g/kg	>5g/kg

Cases of poisoning in children have been reported.
Ingestion of 1 teaspoonful of the oil was fatal for an adult male; the lethal dose for an infant is calculated as a few drops.

Carcinogenesis:
Injections of 15mg in rats for 60-65 weeks induced malignant mesenchymal (connective tissue, blood and lymphatic) tumours similar to those of human malignant fibrous histiocytoma (tumour of phagocytic cells that defend the body against infection).

169 savory oil, summer (Satureja hortensis)	1.37g/kg	0.34g/kg >2.5g/kg guineapigs

NATURAL FRAGRANCE MATERIALS	oral toxicity (rats)	dermal toxicity (rabbits)
170 snakeroot oil (Asarum canadense)	4.48g/kg	>5g/kg
171 Spanish marjoram oil (Thymus mastichina)	>5g/kg	>5g/kg
172 spearmint oil (Mentha spicata)	5g/kg	>5g/kg >2g/kg (guineapigs)
173 spruce oil (Picea mariana & glauca)	>5g/kg	>5g/kg
174 star anise oil (Illicium verum)	2.1-3g/kg	>5g/kg
175 tagetes oil (Tagetes glandulifera/minuta)	3.7g/kg	>5g/kg
176 tangerine oil, expressed (Citrus reticulata)	>5g/kg	>5g/kg
177 tangelo oil, expressed (Citrus reticulata x paradisi)	>5g/kg	>5g/kg
178 tansy oil (Tanacetum vulgare)	1.15g/kg 0.03-0.05g/kg (mice) 0.35g/kg (dogs)	>5g/kg

When administered in increasing amounts, doses twice as large as the toxic dose could be tolerated. The oral toxicity of the main constituent of tansy oil, thujone is 0.3g/kg in rats as compared with 1.15g/kg for the essential oil of tansy. (Essential oils containing large amounts of thujone are poisonous causing convulsions and epileptic-like attacks). Signs of tansy oil poisoning due to thujone include vomiting, gastro-enteritis, flushing, cramps, loss of consciousness, rapid breathing, irregular heartbeat, rigid pupils, uterine bleeding and hepatitis. Death results from circulatory and respiratory arrest and organ degeneration.

179 tarragon oil (Artemisia dracunculus)	1.9ml/kg	>5ml/kg
180 tea tree oil (Melaleuca alternifolia)	1.9g/kg	>5g/kg

NATURAL FRAGRANCE MATERIALS	oral toxicity (rats)	dermal toxicity (rabbits)
181 Texas cedarwood oil (Juniperus mexicana)	>5g/kg	>5g/kg
182 thuja leaf oil (Thuja occidentalis)	0.83g/kg	4.1g/kg
183 thyme oil, red (Thymus vulgaris)	4.7g/kg	>5g/kg
184 tobacco leaf absolute (Nicotiana affinis)	>5g/kg	>5g/kg
185 Tolu balsam (Myroxylon balsamum) *not tested for phototoxicity*	>5g/kg	>5g/kg
186 tonka absolute (Dipteryx odorata)	1.38g/kg	1.26g/kg
187 treemoss concrete (Usnea barbata)	4.33ml/kg	>5g/kg

Lichens appear to be non-toxic to reindeer and other animals who consume large amounts in their normal diet.

188 turmeric oil (Curcuma longa)	>5g/kg	>5g/kg

Powdered turmeric corresponding to 35 times the maximium daily human consumption at 2.5g/kg fed to monkeys did not cause any abnormal effects on body and relative organ weight or gross pathology of the liver, kidneys or heart.

189 vanilla tincture (Vanilla planifolia) *not tested for phototoxicity*	>5g/kg	>2g/kg
190 verbena absolute (Lippia citriodora)	>5g/kg	>5g/kg
191 verbena oil (Lippia citriodora)	>5g/kg	5g/kg >5g/kg (guineapigs)

**French verbena oil tested at 100% produced phototoxic reactions. Not phototoxic at 12.5%.
Moroccan verbena oil tested at 100% produced phototoxic reactions and also irritation. Not phototoxic at 50% but still irritating.**

NATURAL FRAGRANCE MATERIALS	oral toxicity (rats)	dermal toxicity (rabbits)
192 vetivert oil (Vetiveria zizanoides)	>5g/kg	>5g/kg
193 violet leaf absolute (Viola odorata)	not tested	not tested
194 Virginian cedarwood oil (Juniperus virginiana)	>5g/kg	>5g/kg

Use followed by exposure to various rays is sometimes the cause of dermatitis. Pigmentation may follow topical application.

195 wormwood oil (Artemisia absinthium)	0.96g/kg	>5g/kg
196 ylang-ylang oil (Cananga odorata)	>5g/kg	>5g/kg

Chapter 6

Irritation and Sensitisation Reactions of Natural Fragrance Materials on Contact with Human Skin

Testing for skin irritation and sensitisation reactions is carried out with healthy human volunteers. The number of volunteers used in the testing ranges from 19 for gurjun balsam to 30 for myrtle oil, but usually 25 volunteers are used for most of the fragrance materials. Sometimes more volunteers are used: 33 for davana oil and lavandin absolute and 43 for orris absolute. With some of the absolutes and balsams even more volunteers are used in the tests, 50 for copaiba and peru balsams, 52 for verbena absolute and 53 for myrrh absolute, 59 for galbanum oil, and 61 for mastic absolute.

As the task of testing every member of the population would be practically impossible, test procedures were selected to provide a representation of the population. The number of test volunteers used was calculated to produce results for an acceptable percentage of the rest of the population.

A substance tested on 25 randomly selected individuals in the United States without producing any sensitisation reactions cannot mean that the substance is proven to be incapable of sensitising the rest of the 200 million members of the population.

Tests conducted on 25 volunteers with no positive reactions is only reliable for a projected 89% of the population. The tested substance may be safe for the whole population but if it still possesses an adverse potential for the remaining population, this uncertainty is reduced to 11% and below, for which the tests are unable to offer any reliable indications. Using 50 volunteers increases the percentage to 94%. Negative results from using 100 test volunteers reflect a safety projection for 97% of the population. From 200 volunteers, the projection is 98.5% and from 300 test volunteers, 99%. [Saunders 1976]

The number of test volunteers is considered to be adequate at 25 for most of the fragrance materials tested, as a sample representation of the population.

Preparations of the fragrance materials are diluted in petrolatum (a greasy residue from petroleum used as a jelly in pharmacy for medicaments) at percentages calculated at 10 times greater than the maximum concentration used in perfumes.

Testing for primary irritation is conducted by applying the diluted fragrance material on a patch of skin (usually on the forearm or back) under occlusion with cotton gauze for 24-48 hours, after which the patch is removed and the skin examined for indications of a reaction.

Testing for sensitisation is conducted with a similar initial application as for the irritation test, and continued with repeated examination of the skin patch over several days. After an interval of 1-2 weeks, a repeat test is conducted on the same skin patch with the same fragrance material. The skin is then examined for a reaction.

Whenever possible, patients with dermatosis (skin disease) are also tested.

NATURAL FRAGRANCE MATERIALS	% used in in perfume preparations	% tested without irritation/sensitisation in human volunteers
001 ale oil (Pinus sp.)	0.5-3.6	20.0
002 almond oil, bitter (Prunus amygdalus) **Dermatitis in sensitive people has been linked to oil of bitter almond.**	0.04-0.4	4.0
003 almond oil, bitter (Prunus amygdalus) [FFPA]	0.04-0.4	4.0
004 ambrette seed oil (Hibiscus abelmoschus)	0.02-0.12	1.0
005 amyris oil (Amyris balsamifera) [acetylated]	0.54-1.5	10.0
006 angelica root oil (Angelica archangelica)	0.02-0.12	1.0
007 angelica seed oil (Angelica archangelica)	0.02-0.12	1.0
008 anise oil (Pimpinella anisum) **Not a primary irritant to normal human skin but several cases of sensitisation have been reported causing dermatitis, consisting of erythema, desquamation and vesiculation.**	0.054-0.25	2.0
009 armoise oil (Artemisia vulgaris)	0.1-1.2	12.0
010 basil oil, sweet (Ocimum basilicum) *not tested for sensitisation*	0.09-0.4	4.0
011 bay oil (Pimenta racemosa) *not tested for sensitisation*	0.09-1.5	10.0

NATURAL FRAGRANCE MATERIALS	% used in in perfume preparations	% tested without irritation/sensitisation in human volunteers
012 benzoin resinoid (Styrax benzoin)	0.27-0.8	8.0*

* Did not produce any irritation reactions when tested at 8% and is not itself a sensitiser.

Tincture of benzoin that also contains storax and balsams Peru and Tolu has been reported to cause sensitisation from cross-sensitisation to the 2 balsams. In the concentrations and forms employed in toilet preparations, it is not a primary irritant and there is no evidence that it is a sensitiser.

013 bergamot oil, expressed (Citrus bergamia)	0.2-3.0	30.0

not tested for irritation

014 bergamot oil, rectified (Citrus bergamia)	no value	30.0

not tested for irritation

015 birch tar oil (Betula pendula)	0.02-0.2	2.0

An occasional individual may be hypersensitive to birch tar oil.

016 sweet birch oil (Betula lenta)	0.08-0.4	4.0
017 bois de rose oil (Aniba rosaeodora)	0.4-1.0	5.0

Did not produce any irritation or sensitisation reactions when tested at 100% under occlusion on a subject with perfume dermatitis.

018 bois de rose oil (Aniba rosaeodora) [acetylated]	0.4-1.2	12.0
019 boldo leaf oil (Peumus boldus)	0.1-0.4	4.0
020 Brazilian sassafras (Ocotea cymbarum)	0.2-0.8	20.0
021 cabreuva oil (Murocarpus frondosus & fastigiatus)	0.3-0.6	6.0

NATURAL FRAGRANCE MATERIALS	% used in in perfume preparations	% tested without irritation/sensitisation in human volunteers
022 cade tar oil, rectified (Juniperus oxycedrus)	0.04-0.2	2.0

Reported to have slight local activity as an allergen.

023 cajeput oil (Melaleuca leucodendron)	0.04-0.4	4.0
024 calamus oil (Acorus calamus)	0.04-0.4	4.0

Did not produce any sensitisation reactions when tested on 200 consecutive dermatitis patients, and 50 patients sensitive to peru balsam, wood tars, colophony and turpentine. However, dermatitis has been reported in hypersensitive individuals, and when used in bath preparations has been reported to cause skin erythema.

025 camphor oil, white (Cinnamomum camphora)	0.04-0.4	20.0
026 camphor oil, yellow (Cinnamomum camphora)	0.04-0.4	4.0
027 camphor oil, brown (Cinnamomum camphora)	0.04-0.4	4.0
028 cananga oil (Cananga odorata)	0.2-0.8	10.0
029 caraway oil (Carum carvi)	0.02-0.4	4.0
030 cardamom oil (Elettaria cardamomum)	0.04-0.4	4.0
031 carrot seed oil (Daucus carota)	0.04-0.4	4.0

Did not produce any irritation or sensitisation reactions when tested at 100% under occlusion on a subject with perfume dermatitis.

032 cascarilla oil (Croton eluteria)	0.04-0.4	4.0

NATURAL FRAGRANCE MATERIALS	% used in in perfume preparations	% tested without irritation/sensitisation in human volunteers
033 cassia oil (Cinnamomum cassia)	0.05-0.4	4.0*

* Did not produce any irritation reactions when tested at 4% on 25 test volunteers but produced 2 sensitisation reactions. Tested at 100% for 24 hours on 24 human volunteers, produced 2 irritating reactions. Listed as a sensitiser.

034 cedarwood oil, Atlas (Cedrus atlantica)	0.2-0.8	8.0
035 celery seed oil (Apium graveolens)	0.04-0.4	4.0
036 chamomile oil, German (Matricaria chamomilla)	0.04-0.4	4.0
037 chamomile oil, Roman (Anthemis nobilis)	0.04-0.4	4.0
038 chenopodium oil (Chenopodium ambrosioides)	0.04-0.4	4.0
039 cinnamon bark oil (Cinnamomum zeylanicum)	0.09-0.8	8.0*

* Did not produce any irritation reactions when tested at 8% on 25 test volunteers but produced 20 sensitisation reactions. 3 cases reported of acute contact sensitivity to cinnamon oil used in a dentrifice.

040 cinnamon leaf oil (Cinnamomum zeylanicum)	0.1-0.8	10.0
041 citronella oil (Cymbopogon nardus)	0.2-0.8	8.0

In perfumes, considered as a primary irritant and sensitiser. Cases of contact hypersensitivity have been reported resulting in papulovesicular eczema of the fingers, hands and forearms and acneform folliculitis (inflammation of the hair follicles).

042 clove bud oil (Eugenia caryophyllata)	0.2-0.7	5.0

Did not produce any irritation when tested at 2% on normal subjects, and at 0.2% on patients with dermatosis. Tested at 20% in an ointment on 25 human subjects produced 2 primary irritation reactions (erythema). Used in the treatment of dental cavities, damaged the dental pulp and did not promote the development of irritation dentine.

043 clove leaf oil (Eugenia caryophyllata)	0.3-1.0	5.0

NATURAL FRAGRANCE MATERIALS	% used in in perfume preparations	% tested without irritation/sensitisation in human volunteers
044 clove stem oil (Eugenia caryophyllata)	0.2-1.0	10.0

Did not produce any irritation when tested at 2% on normal subjects, and at 0.2% on patients with dermatosis.
Tested at 20% in an ointment on 25 human subjects produced 2 primary irritation reactions (erythema).
Used in the treatment of dental cavities, damaged the dental pulp and did not promote the development of irritation dentine.

045 cognac oil, green (Vitis vinifera)	0.04-0.2	4.0
046 copaiba balsam (Copaifera reticulata)	0.2-0.8	8.0
047 copaiba oil (Copaifera reticulata)	0.2-0.8	8.0
048 coriander oil (Coriandrum sativum)	0.04-0.6	6.0
049 cornmint oil (Mentha arvensis)	0.2-0.8	8.0
050 costus root absolute & concrete (Saussurea lappa)	0.05-0.4	4.0*

* Both costus root absolute and concrete did not produce any irritation reactions when tested at 4% for 48 hours but
- costus root concrete produced 6 sensitisation reactions in 21 test volunteers
- costus root absolute produced 18 sensitisation reactions in 24 test volunteers

051 costus root oil (Saussurea lappa)	0.05-0.4	4.0*

* Did not produce any irritation reactions when tested at 4% for 48 hours but produced sensitisation reactions in all 25 test volunteers, very severely in 8 of them. Tested at 2% in 26 test volunteers, costus oil produced 16 sensitisation reactions.

052 cubeb oil (Piper cubeba)	0.2-0.8	8.0
053 cumin oil (Cuminum cyminum)	0.05-0.4	4.0
054 cypress oil (Cupressus sempervirens)	0.2-1.0	5.0

NATURAL FRAGRANCE MATERIALS	% used in in perfume preparations	% tested without irritation/sensitisation in human volunteers
055 davana oil (Artemisia pallens)	0.08-0.4	4.0
056 deertongue absolute (Liatris odoratissima)	0.08-0.5	5.0
057 deertongue incolore (Liatris odoratissima)	0.04-0.5	5.0
058 dill herb oil (Anethum graveolens)	0.04-0.4	4.0
059 dill seed oil, Indian (Anethum sowa)	0.08-0.4	4.0
060 Douglas fir balsam (Pseudotsuga taxifolia)	0.2-0.8	8.0
061 eau de brouts absolute (Citrus aurantium)	0.04-0.4	4.0
062 elecampane/alantroot oil (Inula helenium)	0.08-0.4	4.0*

* Did not produce any irritation reactions when tested at 4% in 25 test volunteers but produced 23 extremely severe allergic (sensitisation) reactions. Tested on subjects previously sensitised to costus oil, produced severe cross-sensitisation responses.

063 elemi oil (Canarium commune)	0.1-0.6	4.0
064 (Eucalyptus globulus) oil	0.1-1.0	10.0

Did not produce any irritation reactions when retested at 100% for 24 hours, but hypersensitivity has been reported.

065 (Eucalyptus citriodora) oil	(1.0)	10.0
066 (Eucalyptus citriodora) oil [acetylated]	(1.0)	10.0

NATURAL FRAGRANCE MATERIALS	% used in in perfume preparations	% tested without irritation/sensitisation in human volunteers
067 fennel seed oil, bitter (Foeniculum vulgare)	0.04-0.4	4.0*

*Tested at 4% dilution, a pure sample produced no sensitisation reaction. An earlier test using a sample that had deteriorated due to atmospheric oxidation caused sensitisation reactions in 3 of the 25 test volunteers.

068 fennel seed oil, sweet (Foeniculum vulgare)	0.08-0.4	4.0
069 fenugreek absolute (Trigonella foenum-graecum)	0.04-0.2	2.0
070 fig leaf absolute (Ficus carica)	0.08-0.5	? *

* Tested at 5% on 25 subjects, produced 1 irritation reaction and 2 sensitisation reactions.

071 fir cone oil, silver (Abies alba)	0.5-2.0	20.0
072 fir needle oil, silver (Abies alba)	0.5-2.0	20.0
073 fir balsam, Canadian (Abies balsamea)	0.05-0.2	2.0
074 fir needle oil, Canadian (Abies balsamea)	0.1-1.0	10.0
075 fir needle oil, Siberian (Abies sibirica)	0.1-0.25	2.5*

* Did not produce any sensitisation reactions when tested at 2.5% but produced a mild irritation.

076 flouve oil (Anthoxanthum odoratum)	0.04-0.4	4.0

Extracts of the juice of whole grass (but not of the pollen) produced a positive reaction in a subject with summer asthmas.

077 foin absolute (Anthoxanthum odoratum)	0.04-0.3	4.0

NATURAL FRAGRANCE MATERIALS	% used in in perfume preparations	% tested without irritation/sensitisation in human volunteers
078 galbanum oil (Ferula galbaniflua)	0.08-0.7	4.0

Did not produce any primary irritation reactions when tested at 0.1% on 118 dermatosis patients.

079 galbanum resin (Ferula galbaniflua)	(0.8)	8.0

**Did not produce any irritation reactions when tested at 2-20% on normal subjects, and at 0.1% on dermatosis patients.
Tested on a patient who developed contact dermatitis followed by non-eczematous exanthem (eruption) to benzoin tincture, galbanum resin produced cross-sensitisation reactions.**

080 genet absolute (Spartium junceum)	0.04-0.2	12.0
081 geranium oil, Algerian (Pelargonium graveolens)	0.3-1.0	10.0

Did not produce any irritation tested at 20% on normal subjects, and at 2% on dermatosis patients.

082 geranium oil, Bourbon (Pelargonium graveolens)	0.3-1.0	10.0

Geranium leaves have been reported to produce vesicular dermatitis, and the oil may produce dermatitis in hypersensitive individuals.

083 geranium oil, Moroccan (Pelargonium graveolens)	0.3-1.0	10.0
084 ginger oil (Zingiber officinale)	0.08-0.4	4.0

Preparations containing ginger oil may produce dermatitis in hypersensitive individuals.

085 grapefruit oil, expressed (Citrus paradisi)	0.5-1.0	10.0

Did not produce any irritation reactions when retested at 100% for 24 hours.

086 guaiacwood oil (Bulnesia sarmienti)	0.3-0.8	8.0

NATURAL FRAGRANCE MATERIALS	% used in in perfume preparations	% tested without irritation/sensitisation in human volunteers
087 gurjun balsam (Dipterocarpus turbinatus & tuberculatus)	0.1-1.2	12.0
088 gurjun oil (Dipterocarpus turbinatus & tuberculatus)	0.1-0.8	8.0
089 hibawood oil (Thujopsis dolabrata)	0.16-1.2	12.0
090 ho leaf oil (Cinnamomum camphora)	0.2-1.0	10.0
091 honeysuckle absolute (Lonicera caprifolium)	(0.3)	3.0
092 hyacinth absolute (Hyacinthus orientalis)	0.04-0.4	8.0

The juice of hyacinth bulbs has powerful skin-irritating properties, with reported cases of generalised eczema covering almost the entire skin, and dry, scaly and fissured lesions at the fingertips with itching behind both ears.
Dermatoses produced by handling hyacinth bulbs have been reported among sorters and packers in nursery gardens.

093 hyssop oil (Hyssopus officinalis)	0.08-0.4	4.0
094 immortelle absolute (Helichrysum angustifolium)	0.04-0.3	2.0
095 immortelle oil (Helichrysum angustifolium)	0.08-0.4	4.0
096 jasmine absolute (Jasminum officinale)	0.1-0.3	3.0
097 jonquil absolute (Narcissus jonquilla)	0.04-0.2	2.0
098 juniper berry oil (Juniperus communis)	0.1-0.8	8.0

Tested at 100% for 24 hours on 20 human volunteers, produced 2 irritation reactions.

NATURAL FRAGRANCE MATERIALS	% used in in perfume preparations	% tested without irritation/sensitisation in human volunteers
099 juniper oil, Phoenician (Juniperus phoenicia)	(0.1)	1.0
100 karo karounde absolute (Leptactina senegambica)	(0.1)	1.0
101 labdanum/cyste absolute (Cistus ladaniferus)	0.1-0.4	4.0
102 labdanum/cyste oil (Cistus ladaniferus)	0.12-0.8	8.0

Did not produce any irritation or sensitisation reactions when tested at 100% for 48 hours on a subject with perfume dermatitis.

103 laurel leaf oil (Laurus nobilis)	0.04-0.2	2.0

Still did not produce any irritation or sensitisation reactions when retested at 10% in normal subjects, but produced sensitisation reactions in costus oil-sensitised individuals. Contact allergy to laurel leaf oil as topical medicament is common in some European countries, causing hyperaemia and severe inflammation. The allergen in laurel leaf oil has been shown to be an unsaturated ketone.

104 lavandin absolute (Lavandula hybrida)	(1.0)	10.0
105 lavandin oil (Lavandula hybrida)	0.3-1.2	5.0
106 lavandin oil (Lavandula hybrida) [acetylated]	0.03-1.2	10.0
107 lavender absolute (Lavandula officinalis)	0.2-1.0	10.0

Has been listed as a sensitiser.

108 lavender oil (Lavandula officinalis)	0.3-1.2	16.0
109 lavender oil, spike/aspic (Lavandula latifolia)	0.2-0.8	8.0

NATURAL FRAGRANCE MATERIALS	% used in in perfume preparations	% tested without irritation/sensitisation in human volunteers
110 lemon oil, distilled (Citrus limon)	no value	10.0
111 lemon oil, expressed (Citrus limon) Did not produce any irritation reactions when retested at 100% for 24 hours.	0.5-1.0	10.0
112 lemongrass oil, East Indian (Cymbopogon citratus)	0.08-0.7	4.0
113 lemongrass oil, West Indian (Cymbopogon citratus)	0.08-0.7	4.0-5.0
114 lemonmint oil (Mentha citrata)	(0.8)	8.0
115 lime oil, distilled (Citrus aurantifolia) Did not produce any irritation reactions when retested at 100% for 24 hours.	0.4-1.5	15.0
116 lime oil, expressed (Citrus aurantifolia)	0.5-1.5	not tested
117 linaloe wood oil (Bursera delpechiana)	0.4-0.8	8.0
118 litsea oil (Litsea cubeba) Tested at 2% in 2 groups of 200 and 450 dermatitis patients produced 3 and 13 sensitisation reactions respectively.	0.08-0.8	8.0
119 lovage oil (Levisticum officinale) A case of sensitivity to lovage oil has been reported.	0.03-0.2	2.0
120 mace oil (Myristica fragans)	0.12-0.8	8.0

NATURAL FRAGRANCE MATERIALS	% used in in perfume preparations	% tested without irritation/sensitisation in human volunteers
121 mandarin oil, expressed (Citrus reticulata)	(0.8)	8.0
122 marjoram oil (Origanum marjorana)	0.12-0.6	6.0
123 mastic absolute (Pistacia lentiscus)	(0.8)	8.0*

* Did not produce any irritation reactions when tested at 8% on 29 test volunteers, but produced 1 sensitisation reaction; did not produce any sensitisation reactions when retested at 8% in another test group of 32 test volunteers. Pollen extracts did not produce any irritation reactions when tested in non-atopic patients, but when tested on 58 atopic patients produced 16 irritation reactions.

124 mimosa absolute (Acacia decurrens)	0.08-0.1	1.0

May produce dermatitis in hypersensitive individuals.

125 myrrh absolute (Commiphora myrrha)	(0.8)	8.0

Tested in a patient who developed contact dermatitis to benzoin tincture followed by non-eczematous exanthem (eruption), myrrh absolute produced cross-sensitisation reactions.

126 myrrh oil (Commiphora myrrha)	0.16-0.8	8.0
127 myrtle oil (Myrtus communis)	0.04-0.4	4.0
128 narcissus absolute (Narcissus poetieus)	0.04-0.2	2.0

The plant has been reported to be a sensitiser.

129 neroli/orange flower absolute (Citrus aurantium)	0.04-0.3	20.0
130 neroli/orange flower oil (Citrus aurantium)	0.1-0.4	4.0

neroli/orange flower oil is reported to be devoid of irritating properties following at least 20 patch tests with no dermatitis development.

NATURAL FRAGRANCE MATERIALS	% used in in perfume preparations	% tested without irritation/sensitisation in human volunteers
131 nutmeg oil (Myristica fragans)	0.05-0.3	2.0
132 oakmoss concrete (Evernia prunastri)	0.1-0.5	10.0
133 olibanum absolute (Boswellia carterii)	0.1-0.8	8.0
134 olibanum gum (Boswellia carterii)	0.12-0.8	8.0
135 bitter orange oil, expressed (Citrus aurantium)	0.25-1.0	10.0

Cutaneous irritation due to the oil from peeling bitter oranges has been reported, characterised by small vesicular eruptions on the fingers, hands, forearms and face.

136 sweet orange oil, expressed (Citrus sinensis)	0.5-0.8	8.0
137 oregano oil (Origanum vulgare)	0.08-0.2	2.0
138 orris absolute (Iris pallida)	0.04-0.2	3.0

Did not produce any irritation reactions when retested at 100% for 24 hours.

139 palmarosa oil (Cymbopogon martini)	0.3-0.8	8.0
140 parsley herb oil (Petroselinum sativum)	0.04-0.2	2.0
141 parsley seed oil (Petroselinum sativum)	0.04-0.2	2.0

NATURAL FRAGRANCE MATERIALS	% used in in perfume preparations	% tested without irritation/sensitisation in human volunteers
142 patchouli oil (Pogostemon cablin)	0.4-2.0	10.0

Did not produce any irritation reactions when retested at 20% in normal subjects and at 0.1% in patients with dermatosis.

143 pennyroyal oil (Mentha pulegium)	0.12-0.6	6.0
144 pepper oil, black (Piper nigrum)	0.08-0.4	4.0
145 perilla oil (Perilla frutescens)	(0.4)	4.0

Reported to cause various dermal effects to the fingers, such as erosion, fissure, desquamation, thickening or bleeding in half of 152 workers handling perilla plants surveyed. Both the leaves and oil produce allergic reactions in workers with dermatosis.

146 Peru balsam (Myroxylon pereirae)	0.2-0.8	8.0*

* Tested at 8% on 25 test volunteers produced 7 sensitisation reactions.
Reported to be among the most common allergens causing cross-allergic (sensitisation) reactions between Peru balsam and poplar resin.

147 Peru balsam oil (Myroxylon pereirae)	0.1-0.8	8.0
148 Peruvian mastic oil (Schinus molle)	0.1-0.4	4.0
149 petitgrain oil, Bigarade (Citrus aurantium)	(0.8)	8.0

Did not produce any irritation reactions when tested at 0.1% on 48 patients, some with dermatosis.
Tested at 2% on 50 patients sensitised to balsams, produced 2 cross-sensitisation reactions.

150 petitgrain oil, Paraguay (Citrus aurantium)	0.3-0.7	7.0-8.0

Did not produce any irritation reactions when tested at 0.1% in a non-irritating cream base on dermatosis patients.
In 200 consecutive dermatitis patients, 1 sensitisation reaction was reported.

151 petitgrain oil, lemon (Citrus limon)	0.05-0.3	10.0

NATURAL FRAGRANCE MATERIALS	% used in in perfume preparations	% tested without irritation/sensitisation in human volunteers
152 pimento berry oil (Pimenta officinalis)	0.3-1.2	8.0
153 pimento leaf oil (Pimenta officinalis)	0.2-1.2	12.0
154 pine oil, pumilo (Pinus pumilo)	0.2-1.2	12.0*

* Tested at 12% on 22 human volunteers produced 3 irritation reactions but did not produce any sensitisation reactions.

155 pine oil, yarmor (Pinus palustris)	0.2-1.2	12.0
156 pine oil, Scots (Pinus sylvestris)	0.2-1.2	12.0
157 rose absolute, French (Rosa centifolia)	0.1-0.2	2.0
158 rose oil, Bulgarian (Rosa damascena)	0.005-0.2	2.0
159 rose oil, Moroccan (Rosa centifolia)	0.05-0.2	2.0
160 rose oil, Turkish (Rosa damascena)	0.05-0.2	2.0
161 rosemary oil (Rosmarinus officinalis)	0.2-1.0	10.0
162 rue oil (Ruta graveolens)	0.04-0.15	1.0

May harm the mucous membranes and irritate the skin, producing erythema and vesication after frequent dermal contact

NATURAL FRAGRANCE MATERIALS	% used in in perfume preparations	% tested without irritation/sensitisation in human volunteers
163 sage oil, clary French (Salvia sclarea)	0.12-0.8	8.0

Cases of dermatitis have been reported. Positive patch tests have been obtained from the mucous membranes but not from the skin.

164 sage oil, clary Russian (Salvia sclarea)	0.2-0.8	8.0
165 sage oil, Dalmatian (Salvia officinalis)	0.2-0.8	8.0

Retested at 100% for 24 hours in 20 human volunteers produced 1 irritation reaction.

166 sage oil, Spanish (Salvia lavandulaefolia)	0.2-0.8	8.0
167 sandalwood oil (Santalum album)	0.3-1.0	10.0
168 sassafras oil (Sassafras albidum)	0.2-0.4	4.0

Did not produce cross-sensitisation in patients previously reacting to peru balsam, turpentine and colophony.

169 savory oil, summer (Satureja hortensis)	0.1-0.6	6.0
170 snakeroot oil (Asarum canadense)	0.1-0.4	4.0
171 Spanish marjoram oil (Thymus mastichina)	0.12-0.6	6.0
172 spearmint oil (Mentha spicata)	0.08-0.4	4.0

Reported case of allergic stomatitis and dermatitis provoked by spearmint oil in toothpaste

173 spruce oil (Picea mariana & glauca)	(0.1)	1.0

Tested at 20% for 48 hours in 1247 human volunteers produced 62 sensitisation reactions.

NATURAL FRAGRANCE MATERIALS	% used in in perfume preparations	% tested without irritation/sensitisation in human volunteers
174 star anise oil (Illicium verum)	0.08-0.4	4.0
175 tagetes oil (Tagetes glandulifera/minuta)	0.08-0.2	2.0

Reported to cause primary irritation and severe and prolonged allergic contact dermatitis in humans following exposure to the fresh leaves and flowers. Did not produce cross-sensitisation in patients previously sensitised to costus absolute.

176 tangerine oil, expressed (Citrus reticulata)	0.1-0.5	5.0
177 tangelo oil, expressed (Citrus reticulata x paradisi)	0.2-0.8	8.0
178 tansy oil (Tanacetum vulgare)	0.12-0.4	4.0
179 tarragon oil (Artemisia dracunculus)	0.04-0.4	4.0
180 tea tree oil (Melaleuca alternifolia)	(0.1)	1.0
181 Texas cedarwood oil (Juniperus mexicana)	0.2-0.8	8.0

Reported to be a slight acute or chronic local irritant and allergen.

182 thuja leaf oil (Thuja occidentalis)	0.2-0.4	4.0
183 thyme oil, red (Thymus vulgaris)	0.05-0.8	8.0
184 tobacco leaf absolute (Nicotiana affinis)	0.004-0.04	1.0

NATURAL FRAGRANCE MATERIALS	% used in in perfume preparations	% tested without irritation/sensitisation in human volunteers
185 Tolu balsam (Myroxylon balsamum)	0.1-0.2	2.0

Did not produce any irritation or sensitisation reactions when tested at 100% for 48 hours in a patient with perfume dermatitis.

Trial with 67 patients allergic to Peru balsam -
Tested at 5% as powder in vaseline produced 21% positive reactions
Tested at 10% in alcohol produced 50% positive reactions
Tested at 1% in alcohol produced 73% positive reactions
Positive reactions were more frequent with alcoholic solution.

Sensitivity to Tolu balsam is always accompanied by sensitivity to Peru balsam and benzoin and the constituents coniferyl benzoate and coniferyl cinnamate.

186 tonka absolute (Dipteryx odorata)	0.08-0.8	8.0
187 treemoss concrete (Usnea barbata)	0.1-0.5	10.0
188 turmeric oil (Curcuma longa)	0.2-0.4	4.0
189 vanilla tincture (Vanilla planifolia)	0.2-1.0	10.0

Did not produce any primary irritation when tested at 100% on 31 human volunteers
Tested on 73 patients sensitive to Peru balsam produced 34 cross-sensitisation reactions,
however patients sensitive to vanilla tincture did not suffer from sensitisation reactions when tested with Peru balsam.

190 verbena absolute (Lippia citriodora)	no value	12.0*

* Did not produce any irritation reactions when tested at 12% in 26 test volunteers but produced 3 sensitisation reactions.
Did not produce any sensitisation reactions when retested at 2%

191 verbena oil (Lippia citriodora)	(1.2)	?*

* Tested at 12% for 48 hours (using 6 different samples) on 159 human volunteers produced 3 irritation reactions;
* Tested at 12% on different panels of 25 human volunteers -
French verbena oil produced 13 sensitisation reactions
Grasse verbena oil produced 15 sensitisation reactions
Moroccan verbena oil produced 4 sensitisation reactions
Boufarik verbena oil produced no sensitisation reactions in 30 test volunteers
2 samples of pure verbena oil of unknown origin -
tested on 159 volunteers produced 1 irritation reaction each and
tested on 28 volunteers produced 2 and 18 sensitisation reactions

NATURAL FRAGRANCE MATERIALS	% used in in perfume preparations	% tested without irritation/sensitisation in human volunteers
192 vetivert oil (Vetiveria zizanoides)	0.3-0.8	8.0
193 violet leaf absolute (Viola odorata)	0.04-0.2	2.0
194 Virginian cedarwood oil (Juniperus virginiana)	0.2-0.8	8.0
195 wormwood oil (Artemisia absinthium)	0.08-0.25	2.0
196 ylang-ylang oil (Cananga odorata)	0.3-1.0	10.0

Chapter 7

Grading of Fragrance Materials including IFRA recommendations

The natural fragrance materials tested by the RIFM were selected for their importance in perfumery. They total 196 in number and consist of the following:

Group I	Group II	Group III
140 distilled essential oils	28 absolutes	1 gum
9 expressed essential oils	2 concretes	1 resin
	1 incolore	6 balsams
	1 tincture	
	1 resinoid	

2 spurious essential oils & 4 modified fragrance materials

The primary requirement for the selection of fragrance materials by the RIFM for testing is a practical one. Selected materials are required to be representative of materials in actual use in the fragrance industry. They do not always conform to botanical precision. The few test materials that are defined by their commercially accepted name rather than by their correct botanical nature will be indicated.

Values for the toxicity testing are measured either in volume - millilitre(ml) or in weight - gram(g). Having a density of 1, water will weigh exactly 1 g for 1 ml. The fragrance materials have different densities, most essential oils being lighter than water. However the difference is not great, and for convenience, all conversions will be referred to in mls.

The values for both oral and dermal toxicity are calculated at an upper limit of 5ml of the tested material per kg of body weight. If the value derived from the test animals is assumed to correspond to humans, this value would be the theoretical equivalent of 350ml as the toxic dose for an adult weighing 70kg. Most of the tested fragrance materials are of low toxicity requiring quantities greater than 350mls to cause toxicity. Values for the few materials that have higher toxicity will be indicated. The theoretical adult toxic dose can be calculated by simply multiplying by 70.

All the fragrance materials included in this book comply with the U.S. Code of Federal Regulations (21CFR 101.22a3) definition as a natural flavouring substance. With few exceptions, most are considered by the U.S. Food Extracts Manufacturer's Association (FEMA) as having GRAS (generally regarded as safe) status. Subsequently they are also included in the approved lists of either one or both the U.S. Food and Drug Administration (FDA) and the Council of Europe. Some less commonly used materials have not yet been included while a few are not considered sufficiently safe to be included. These will also be indicated.

All known hazards when significant will be highlighted and the International Fragrance Association (IFRA) recommendations for safe levels of use will be included regarding that particular hazard or combination of hazards.

The Quenching Effect -
It has been observed during testing that although individual pure compounds, particularly certain aldehydes, isolated from a natural source proved to be strong sensitisers, the essential oils from which they were isolated did not induce sensitisation even when the specific aldehydes were present in concentrations as high as 85%. It appears that other components in the natural essential oils, particularly terpenes and alcohols, inhibited the induction of sensitisation. This phenomenon is recognised as the quenching effect. Quenching seems to be a consistent behaviour of natural essential oils. Therefore just because an essential oil contains compounds that have been shown to be hazardous, the essential oil is not necessarily hazardous itself.

Recommendations for safe use are usually within a range of values, depending on whether the fragrance material is used on its own or in combination with other materials. When the recommended values provided in this chapter are different from the IFRA values, the upper values account for the quenching effect when the material is used in combination.

Some additional information on chemical composition has also been included in this chapter. Since qualified aromatherapists will already be familiar with the chemical composition of the more commonly used essential oils, having learnt about them during their professional training, information on composition will be limited to fragrance materials that are toxicologically or otherwise significant or that are obscure or less well known. Some background information will aslo be provided for these materials.

Group I - Essential Oils

This group of essential oils includes all those extracted by distillation (140) plus the citrus essential oils that are extracted by expression (9). They are divided into 15 grades according to the combined hazards of each individual oil.

Grade 1 -
This is the safest category of essential oils, all having an oral and dermal toxicity of about or above 350mls for a 70kg adult. They are further divided into groups at the different percentages at which they were tested without producing any irritation or sensitisation reactions in human volunteers. The few that were retested pure at 100% without producing either adverse reaction will be indicated. All these essential oils were tested and shown not to be phototoxic in any significant way unless otherwise stated. (**65 essential oils**)

Grade 2 -
This category is comparable to Grade I in every way except that their dermal toxicity appears to be twice that of their oral toxicity. (**10 essential oils**)

Grade 3 -
This is the category for the expressed citrus essential oils. Their extraction by expression allows for non-volatile components to render some of them phototoxic. None of the citrus oils extracted by distillation have this problem and they are included in the Grade 1 category. (**9 essential oils**)

Grades 4 to 7 -
The essential oils from Grades 4 to 7 have increasing degrees of oral toxicity.

Grade 4 - oral toxicity at over 3.5g/kg to under 4.5g/kg (**9 essential oils**)

Grade 5 - oral toxicity at over 2.5g/kg to under 3.5g/kg (**11 essential oils**)

Grade 6 - oral toxicity at over 1.5g/kg to under 2.5g/kg (**8 essential oils**)

Grade 7 - oral toxicity at over 0.5g/kg to under 1.5g/kg (**5 essential oils**)

However all of the essential oils from these four grades have low dermal toxicity comparable to the grade 1 essential oils at 350mls for a 70kg adult.

Grade 1 to 7 essential oils are generally non-hazardous for skin applications.

Essential oils with potential hazards.

Grade 8 -
This is a category of high oral toxicity at less than 0.5/kg corresponding to a theoretical toxic dose of 35g for a 70kg adult. When the oral toxicity of a material is determined to be below 0.5g/kg, the dermal toxicity value is no longer considered separately even when shown to be safe. (**3 essential oils**)

Grade 9 -
This is a category for irritation potential. The essential oils included were shown to exhibit moderate irritation. (**6 essential oils**)

Grade 10 -
This category includes essential oils that are extracted by distillation and yet exhibit severe phototoxic potential. (**2 essential oils**)

Grade 11 -
This is a category for essential oils that exhibit both sensitisation and phototoxic potentials. (**1 essential oil**)

Grade 12 -
This is a category for sensitisation potential. The essential oils included were shown to exhibit moderate to severe sensitisation. (**4 essential oils**)

Grade 13 -
This category includes essential oils that were shown to be significantly more dermally toxic than the Grade 1 essential oils. (**7 essential oils**)

Grade 14 -
This is a category for carcinogenic potential. It includes the few essential oils that contain components shown in experiments to be able to induce tumours in test animals. However the essential oils themselves exhibit anticarcinogenic actions. (**5 essential oils**)

Grade 15 -
This is the most hazardous category of all the essential oils tested. It includes the few essential oils with very high oral and dermal toxicity. (**4 essential oils**)

Grade 8 to 15 essential oils possess certain hazards and appropriate caution regarding their use are recommended. These recommendations will be found in their corresponding sections.

Group I Grade 1 - very low toxicity and hazard potential

tested from 12-30% on human volunteers without any irritation or sensitisation reactions

bergamot oil, rectified (Citrus bergamia) Rutaceae - 30%
lime oil, distilled (Citrus aurantifolia) Rutaceae - 15%

Natural expressed bergamot and lime oils contain non-volatile components including furocoumarins such as bergapten and oxypeucedanin which are phototoxic, bergamot and lime oils being the two most phototoxic of all the citrus oils.

Human skin treated with expressed bergamot oil in a suntan lotion and cologne and exposed to the sun suffers from a pronounced and fairly permanent spotting and pigmentation, but applied in a cream in the absence of light, gives excellent results on skin damaged by bacteria or fungi. [Minerva Med (1952) 43/780]

Eleven cases of photodermatitis due to expressed lime oil (Persian) have been reported and a photodynamic reaction was experimentally produced by expressed lime oil on the skin and subsequent solar irradiation. [Archs Derm Syph (1941) 44/571]

When bergamot oil is rectified under vacuum, the non-volatile components including the furocoumarins are completely removed and the oil becomes furocoumarin free (FCF) and non-phototoxic.

Distilled lime oil is not irritating to human skin at up to 100% when tested for up to 24 hours.

camphor oil, white (Cinnamomum camphora) Lauraceae- 20%
[not tested for phototoxicity]

The biochemistry of the camphor tree is very complex and continues to maintain biochemical intrigue. Camphor oil is usually extracted from the Japanese camphor tree. The Taiwanese camphor tree occurs as 5 main chemotypes: eucamphor chemotype (50% camphone), cineola chemotype (76% 1,8-cineole), safrola chemotype (80% safrole), linaloola chemotype (80% linalool) and sesquiterpena chemotype (40-60% nerolidol). Crude camphor oil is fractionated into white, yellow and brown camphor oils. A blue camphor oil is also available containing a- & b- bisabolol, t-cadinol, cubenol, t-muurolol, junenol, nerolidol, cadinenol and epicubenol. [Perfumer & Flavourist (1976) Vol.1 No.4 pgs.31]

Camphor oil, white is rich in cineole and is the fraction that is suitable for aromatherapy use as the yellow and brown fractions have a very high content of safrole, which is hazardous.

The symptoms of camphor oil poisoning by ingestion include nausea, vomiting, colic, headache, dizziness, delirium, muscle twitching, epileptiform convulsions, depression of the central nervous system and coma. Breathing is difficult and anuria may occur. Death from respiratory failure is rare though fatalities in children have been recorded from ingesting 1g of camphor oil. [Martindale's Extra-Pharmacopoeia 28th ed. 1982]

Poisoning usually occurs from administration of camphorated oil to children in mistake for castor oil. Of 175 admissions of children aged from 6 months to 5 years to the Newcastle General Hospital for poisoning, 10 related to the ingestion of camphorated oil.
[Br med J (1973) 1/803]

A 77 year old man who ingested 60 ml of camphorated oil developed vomiting and convulsions. He recovered following treatment by haemodialysis with 8 litres of soya oil for 4.5 hours to remove 6.56g of camphor from his system. [H.E. Ginn, J Am med Ass (1968) 203/230]

A man who attempted suicide by the ingestion of 150 ml of camphorated oil suffered peripheral circulatory shock, severe dehydration due to vomiting, and 3 attacks of severe and prolonged grand mal epilepsy. He recovered after intensive supportive treatment. The dose of camphor was believed to be one of the highest to be followed by survival.
[R.H. Vasey & S.J. Karayanopoulis, Br med J (1972) 1/112]

Camphorated oil is prepared with 20% camphor in any suitable fixed oil.

The occasional hypersensitive individual may also react adversely to camphor oil applied externally on the skin. **Reduce to 0.1% for hypersensitive individuals**.

Prolonged seizures occurred in a 15 month old child following skin contact with camphor and 1 year later, a brief seizure followed inhalation of a camphor preparation.
[R.R. Skoglund, Clin Pediat (1977) 16/901]

fir cone oil, silver (Abies alba) Pinaceae - 20%
fir needle oil, silver (Abies alba) Pinaceae - 20%
pine oil, Scots (Pinus sylvestris) Pinaceae - 12%
hibawood oil (Thujopsis dolabrata) Cupressaceae -12%

The IFRA recommendations for essential oils obtained from trees of the Pinaceae family is to use only when the level of peroxides is kept to the lowest practicable level, having a peroxide value of less than 10 millimoles peroxide per litre (as determined according to the Essential Oil Association's method). This recommendation is based on the RIFM's test results showing sensitising potentials of essential oils derived from the Pinaceae family containing peroxides.

lavender oil (Lavandula officinalis) Labiatae - 16%

Three types of lavender oil are available commercially and all three can be used in aromatherapy. The true lavender oil is the one mostly used; lavandin oil is more camphoraceous and is also sometimes used; while spike lavender or aspic oil is marginally more toxic than the other two.

lavender oil contains no less than 35% linalyl acetate.
lavandin oil contains 20 - 28% of linalyl acetate.
spike lavender oil contains up to 20% of cineole.

tested at up to 10% on human volunteers without any irritation or sensitisation reactions.

sandalwood oil (Santalum album) Santalaceae

The sandalwood of India has been highly prized since ancient times, enshrined in the poetry and tradition of the Hindus and sandalwood oil has been an item of commerce for decades. However, prior to the first world war, sandalwood was exported to England, Germany and the United States for distillation. Since then sandalwood oil has been distilled locally in India with an annual production of between 2000 - 2500 tons. Sandalwood oil contains up to 90% of santalol. [Perfumer & Flavourist (1981) Vol.6 No.5 pgs.32-4]

Another species of sandalwood occurs in Western Australia. The Australian sandalwood oil (Eucarya spicata) contains up to 80% of santalol and farnesol. It has been shown in tests to be one of the most active essential oils against the gram positive bacteria, Staphylococcus aurens and the yeast, Candida albicans. However at present, the Australian sandalwood tree is a protected species of the Australian government and no Australian sandalwood oil is commercially available until the tree is sufficiently conserved.
[Perfumer & Flavourist (1979) Vol.4 No.2 pgs.23-5]

patchouli oil (Pogostemon cablin) Labiatae

Patchouli oil did not produce any irritation reactions when retested at up to 20% on healthy subjects and at 0.1% on dermatosis patients.

ylang-ylang oil (Cananga odorata) Annonaceae
cananga oil (Cananga odorata) Annonaceae

Cananga oil is similar to ylang-ylang oil. The first distillation of the flowers produces the ylang-ylang oil which has the finest quality. Subsequent distillations of the same flowers are called cananga oils, usually numbered 1,2,3 in decreasing order of quality. Both the ylang-ylang and cananga oils are used in perfumery, but in aromatherapy, only the ylang-ylang oil is used having superior therapeutic properties. Safety applications are comparable for both oils.

rosemary oil (Rosmarinus officinalis) Labiatae

Rosemary like many plants of the Labiatae family occurs as several chemotypes, however, the most commonly used rosemary oil contains up to 50% of cineole. Distilled from the dried leaves, rosemary oil is of great importance to the fragrance industry because of its fresh, herbaceous top notes and its clean, tenacious woody-balsamic dry-out.

fir needle oil, Canadian (Abies balsamea) Pinaceae

Safety application for Canadian fir needle oil is comparable to that of Silver fir needle oil.

lemon oil, distilled (Citrus limon) Rutaceae
petitgrain oil, lemon (Citrus limon) Rutaceae

Lemon petitgrain oil is slightly less toxic than the more commonly used petitgrain oil from bitter orange. However, petitgrain oil from bitter orange is adequate for aromatherapy use.

(Eucalyptus globulus) oil. Myrtaceae [oral toxicity at 4.44g/kg]

Eucalyptus globulus oil has been taken by mouth for catarrh. The symptoms of poisoning are epigastric burning, nausea and vomiting, dizziness and muscular weakness, miosis, tachycardia and a feeling of suffocation. Cyanosis, delirium and convulsions may occur. Death has been recorded from doses varying from 3.5 - 21 ml. [Martindale's Extra-Pharmacopoeia 28th ed. 1982]

Eucalyptus globulus oil is not irritating on human skin at up to 100% when tested for up to 24 hours; however, hypersensitivity has been reported in some individuals.

---

tested at up to 8% on human volunteers without any irritation or sensitisation reactions

lemonmint (Mentha citrata) Labiatae

Lemonmint oil is the least orally toxic from the four species of mint tested, followed by cornmint oil and spearmint oil in increasing order of toxicity, with pennyroyal oil being the most orally toxic of the mints.

sage oil, Spanish (Salvia lavendulaefolia) Labiatae

Spanish sage oil is the least orally toxic from the three species of sage tested, followed by clary sage oil and Dalmation sage oil in increasing order of toxicity.

thyme oil, garden red (Thymus vulgaris) Labiatae [oral toxicity at 4.7g/kg]

Two types of thyme oil are available commercially from the garden thyme (Thymus vulgaris). The red oil is the coloured crude distillate and the white oil is the colourless distillate rectified by redistillation. The NIOSH of the United States concurs with the RIFM on the oral toxicity value of thyme oil, red, at 4.7g/kg; and determined the oral toxicity value of thyme oil, white, at 2.84g/kg implying that the white oil is one and a half times more toxic than the red oil. Both oils are used in aromatherapy.

labdanum oil (Cistus ladaniferus) Cistaceae *[not tested for phototoxicity]*

Tested at 100% on a patient with perfume dermatitis for 48 hours, labdanum oil did not produce any irritation or sensitisation reactions.

palmarosa oil (Cymbopogon martini) Graminae
vetivert oil (Vetiveria zizanoides) Graminae
Vetivert oil is the least hazardous from the aromatic grasses. Palmarosa oil is similar to vetivert oil in toxicity and is the least hazardous among the Cymbopogon species. Safety application is comparable for both oils.

petitgrain oil, Bigarade (Citrus aurantium) Rutaceae
petitgrain oil, Paraguay (Citrus aurantium) Rutaceae
Petitgrain oil is usually distilled from the leaves and twigs of the bitter orange tree, but other citrus trees are also sometimes used. The Bigarade is from Europe, having a long tradition of use; while the Paraguay is from South America, and was introduced more recently. Safety application is comparable for both types of petitgrain oils.

Tested at 0.1% in a non-irritating cream base on 48 patients, some with dermatosis, petitgrain oil did not produce any irritation reactions. However, 1 positive sensitisation reaction was observed in 200 consecutive dermatitis patients. Tested at 2% on 50 patients previously sensitised to balsams, petitgrain oil produced 2 cross-sensitisation reactions. **Reduce to 0.1% for individuals with dermatosis or cross-sensitivity.**

linaloe wood oil (Bursera delpechiana) Burseraceae
Composition: 48% linalool, 40% linalyl acetate, 8.5% a-terpineol, 3.5% geranyl acetate, 2.5% neryl acetate and 2% linalool oxide. May contain up to 8% of sesquiterpene waxes and resins.
[Perfumer & Flavourist (1976) Vol.1 No.1 pgs.1]

guaiac wood oil (Bulnesia sarmienti) Zygophyllaceae
The guaiac wood tree is found in Paraguay and Argentina.
Composition: 40-45% bulnesol, 27-33% guaicol, 4.5% a-bulnesene, 2.5% b-bulnesene, 2% guaioxide, 2.2% 10-epi-g-eudesmol, 1.2% elemol and 0.18% b-eudesmol.
[Perfumer & Flavourist (1992) Vol.17 No.6 pgs.52]

copaiba oil (Copaifera reticulata) Leguminosae *[not tested for phototoxicity]*
Composition: 50% caryophyllene, 15% a-copaene, 7-10% trans-a-bergamotene, 3.6% a-cubenene, 2.4% d-elemene and 1.6% b-elemene. [Perfumer & Flavourist (1980) Vol.5 No.4 pgs.32]

juniper berry oil (Juniperus communis) Cupressaceae
Juniper oil is used as a diuretic but it should not be employed during pregnancy or in the presence of renal disease. [Martindale's Extra-Pharmacopoeia 28th ed. 1982]

Tested at 100% on 20 volunteers for 24 hours, juniper berry oil produced 2 irritation reactions.

cubeb oil (Piper cubeba) Piperaceae

The essential oil of cubeb is steam distilled from the sun-dried fruits (berries) of the cubeb plant, a species of pepper which resembles the black pepper vine. They are both climbing perennials growing in India and Malaysia.

Composition: 11% b-cubenene, 10.4% coapene, 8.8% d-cadinene, 7% a-cubebene, 5% g-humulene, 4.6% sabinene, 4.2% aromadendrene, 3.7% caryophyllene, 3.7% calamenene, 2.2% a-thujene, 1.5% b-bisabolene, 1.2% a-muurolene, 10% cubebol, 3.5% cubenol & epi-cubenol, 3.5% nerolidol, 3.7% cesarone, 2.2% a-terpineol, 0.7% 1,8-cineole and 0.3% apiole.
[Perfumer & Flavourist (1980) Vol.5 No.6 pgs.28]

litsea oil (Litsea cubeba) Lauraceae [dermal toxicity at 4.8g/kg]

The essential oil of litsea is steam distilled from the fruits (berries) of the litsea plant which is a deciduous tree growing to a height of 2.7 metres in the eastern Himalayas and China extending to the island of Taiwan.

Composition: 8.4% limonene, 3% myrcene, 40.6% geranial, 33.8% neral, 4.4% methyl-heptenone, 1.7% linalool, 1.65% linalyl acetate, 1.58% geraniol, 1% nerol and traces of citronellal, citronellol, neryl acetate and geranyl acetate.
[Perfumer & Flavourist (1981) Vol.6 No.3 pgs.47-8]

Tested at 2% litsea oil produced 3 sensitisation reactions in 200 dermatitis patients and 13 sensitisation reactions in another group of 450 dermatitis patients. Litsea oil is not sensitising to healthy individuals. **Reduce to 0.1% for patients with dermatitis.**

gurjun oil (Dipterocarpus turbinatus & tuberculatus) Dipterocarpaceae

The essential oil of gurjun is steam distilled from the balsam. In compounding, it is used to blend with ylang-ylang and patchouli oils.

Composition: 50% a-gurjunene, 15% b-gurjunene (calarene) - identical to d-aristolene, 5% allo-aromadendrene, 5% copaene, 2 - 4% caryophyllene, a-humulene, b-humulene, b-elemene and valencene. (Total sesquiterpene content - 76%).
[Perfumer & Flavourist (1980) Vol.5 No.3 pgs.64]

cedarwood oil, Atlas (Cedrus atlantica) Pinaceae

The Atlas and Himalayan are the only true cedarwoods commercially used for producing essential oils. The oil from the Atlas is more readily available than the Himalayan. Other North American conifers called 'cedarwood', especially the Virginian and Texas, only have fragrances slightly resembling that of the true cedarwoods and are not cedarwoods themselves.

The essential oils of litsea, gurjun and cedarwood are not yet included in the approved lists of both the U.S. Food and Drug Administration and the Council of Europe.

tested at up to 4% on human volunteers without any irritation or sensitisation reactions

chamomile oil, Roman (Anthemis nobilis) Compositae
chamomile oil, German (Matricaria chamomilla) Compositae

Roman and German chamomile oils are very similar in their therapeutic actions, the German oil having a higher content of the anti-inflammatory azulene than the Roman oil. Safety application is comparable for both types of chamomile oil.

Anaphylactic shock has been reported with chamomile tea. Allergic rhinitis may occur in atopic subjects known to be sensitive to pollen. [J Am med Ass (1978) 240/109 & 244/330]

davana oil (Artemisia pallens) Compositae

Davana oil is the least orally toxic from the four species of Artemisia tested, followed by tarragon oil, wormwood oil and armoise oil in increasing order of oral toxicity; armoise oil having comparable oral toxicity to pennyroyal oil.

immortelle oil (Helichrysum angustifolium) Compositae

The immortelle plant, H. angustifolium is also known as H. italicum. The essential oil from this plant is produced in Italy and Yugoslavia. Immortelle oils produced in Spain and France are obtained from H. stoechas. French immortelle oil has a lower ester content than Yugoslavian immortelle oil. Corsican immortelle oil which has the richest ester content (64% neryl acetate) is also available. Immortelle oil from all sources contains b-diketones, responsible for the distinctive earthy, hay-spice odour associated with it.

Composition: a-pinene, b-pinene, camphene, cis-ocimene, trans-ocimene, myrcene, limonene, neryl acetate, linalool, nerol, geraniol, terpinen-4-ol, 1,8-cineole, eugenol with hentriacontane.
No quantitative data was available. [Perfumer & Flavourist (1978) Vol.3 No.5 pgs.25-7]

In addition the Yugoslavian oil contains two b-diketones and the French oil contains three.
Yugoslavian immortelle oil: 3,5-dimethyl-octan-4,6-dione & 2,4-dimethyl-heptan-3,5-dione.
French immortelle oil: 2,5,7-trimethyl-dec-2-en-6,8-dione, 2,5,7,9-tetramethyl-dec-2-en-6,8-dione & 2,5,7,9-tetramethyl-undec-2-en-6,8-dione. [Perfumer & Flavourist (1978) Vol.3 No.1 pgs.55]

myrtle oil (Myrtus communis) Myrtaceae

Test animals (rats) developed a tolerance by an adaptive mechanism to higher doses of myrtle oil when given daily oral doses. At the lethal dose of 7.36ml/kg, death was caused by central nervous system depression.

Peruvian mastic (Schinus molle) Anacardiaceae
The essential oil of Peruvian mastic is pale green to olive green in colour. It is only of minor commercial importance and has a low profile.

Composition: 12.7% a-phellandrene, 11.6% myrcene, 10.5% p-cymene, 9% limonene, 7.2% b-phellandrene, 6% viridiflorol, 4.7% d-cadinene, 3.8% a-cadinene, 3% a-humulene, 3% a-pinene, 2.5% spathulenol, 2.5% cadinol, 2.2% muurolol, 2.1% a-terpinene, 1.5% caryophyllene, 1.3% terpinen-4-ol, 1% a-gurjunene and 1% carvacrol.
[Perfumer & Flavourist (1976) Vol.1 No.5 pgs.14]

Peruvian mastic (Schinus molle) and Brazilian mastic (Schinus terebinthifolius) are both trees that are closely related to the poison ivy (Toxicodendron radicans). The Peruvian mastic was introduced into California in the late 18th century while the Brazilian mastic was introduced into Florida at the end of the 19th century.

Dried fruits of the Peruvian mastic are used as a condiment in South America. They are also used as a substitute for black pepper, having a similar flavour to it. When taken in large quantities, the fruits are toxic, causing gastrointestinal inflammation resulting in severe vomiting and diarrhoea. The fruits of Brazilian mastic are also toxic and known to cause internal compaction and fatal colic in horses that have eaten the green berries. Ingesting 1 - 2 berries in humans produces an initial sweet terpenic taste changing to a warm pleasant sensation in the mouth after 10 minutes. This is quickly followed by a burning sensation in the mouth with a slightly uncomfortable feeling in the stomach, the effect lasting for more than 2 hours. Additionally, animals rubbing against the trunk of the Brazilian mastic tree acquired dermatitis and the aromatic exudate from the wood is known to cause lesions and severe itching in humans. When in bloom, the trees emit an irritant which causes sinus and nasal congestion, eye irritation, sneezing and breathing difficulties.

However the distilled essential oils of both Peruvian mastic and Brazilian mastic, although responsible for the terpenic flavour of the fruits, did not cause any irritation of the mucous membranes or unpleasant effects when ingested in an aqueous dextrose solution (dilution and dosage unspecified). The essential oils of both plants appear to be safe in normal use.
[Perfumer & Flavourist (1984) Vol.9 No.5 pgs.65-9]

cascarilla oil (Croton elutheria) Euphorbiaceae
The essential oil of cascarilla is steam distilled from the dried bark. It is only produced in small amounts annually, obtained mainly from the Bahama Islands. In perfumery, it is important for its power and tenacity when combined with other fragrances.

Composition: a-thujene, camphene, a- & b- pinene, myrcene, limonene, p-myrcene, b-elemene, caryophyllene, cuparene, g-terpinene, calamenene, a-calacorene, linalool, borneol, eugenol, terpinen-4-ol and cascarillediene (sesquiterpene), cascarillic acid and cacarillone (diterpene).
No quantitative data was available. [Perfumer & Flavourist (1977) Vol.2 No.1 pgs.3]

lemongrass oil, E. Indian (Cymbopogon citratus) Graminae
lemongrass oil, W. Indian (Cymbopogon citratus) Graminae
Two types of lemongrass oil are available commercially. One from Asia and another from the Caribbean. Safety application is comparable for both types of lemongrass oil.

cardamom oil (Elettaria cardamomum) Zingiberaceae
turmeric oil (Curcuma longa) Zingiberaceae
2.5g of powdered turmeric corresponding to 35 times the maximum daily human consumption fed to monkeys did not cause any abnormal effects on body and relative organ weight or gross pathology of the liver, kidneys or heart.

ginger oil (Zingiber officinale) Zingiberaceae
pepper oil (Piper nigrum) Piperaceae
Both pepper and ginger possess low-level phototoxicity which is not significant when they are used on their own or with other non-phototoxic essential oils. However, the phototoxic level can increase when they are used with other phototoxic essential oils. Ginger oil may also cause dermatitis in hypersensitive individuals. **Reduce to 0.1% for hypersensitive individuals.**

carrot seed oil (Daucus carota) Umbelliferae
The essential oil of carrot is distilled from the seeds. This oil is different from the expressed carrot root oil which is a fixed oil rich in b-carotene (pro-Vitamin A).

Tested at 100% under occlusion on a patient with perfume dermatitis, carrot seed oil did not produce any irritation or sensitisation reactions.

celery seed oil (Apium graveolens) Umbelliferae
Workers harvesting and preparing celery for canning have been reported to suffer from phototoxic reactions producing blisters and lesions. The dermatitis was confined to the upper limbs and associated with itching apparently caused by contact with the plant oil. However the photoreactive substance producing vesicular and bullous lesions on human skin following exposure to sunlight was found only in pink rot celery. The RIFM test results showed celery oil to be non-phototoxic.

Pink rot is caused by Sclerotinia fungus infecting the celery and subsequently producing the furocoumarins that are responsible for a photosensitising action resulting in skin rashes in humans. The dermatitis that develops on the hands of celery growers is a well recognised condition known as 'celery rash'; this is now thought to result from infection of the celery plants with the fungus Sclerotinia. [United Kingdom Ministry of Agriculture (1984) Reference Book 161 replacing Bulletin 161]

fennel seed oil, bitter (Foeniculum vulgare) Umbelliferae
[oral toxicity at 4.52g/kg]
Tested at 4% on 29 volunteers, fennel seed oil, bitter did not produce any irritation or sensitisation reactions. **(Tests with samples of bitter fennel seed oil that had deteriorated due to atmospheric oxidation causing an increase in the levels of p-cymene above 2% and anisaldehyde above 0.3% produced 3 sensitisation reactions in 25 volunteers).**

dill seed oil, Indian (Anethum sowa) Umbelliferae [oral toxicity at 4.6g/kg]
In the United States, two types of dill are cultivated: the European dill (A. graveolens) from Bulgaria, Hungary or Poland and the Indian dill (A. sowa). Various agronomic and processing conditions are associated with their cultivation. Their essential oils are differentiated by the presence of dill apiole in Indian dill and absence in European dill.
[Perfumer & Flavourist (1977) Vol.2 No.2 pgs.29]

galbanum oil (Ferula galbaniflua) Umbelliferae *[not tested for phototoxicity]*
Tested at 0.1% on 118 dermatosis patients, galbanum oil did not produce any primary irritation reactions.

spearmint oil (Mentha spicata) Labiatae
Spearmint oil has been shown to be safe, applied at up to 4%. However, there has been a reported case of allergic stomatitis and dermatitis provoked by spearmint oil in toothpaste. **Reduce to 0.1% for hypersensitive individuals.**

neroli/orange flower oil (Citrus aurantium) Rutaceae
[oral toxicity at 4.5g/kg]
Neroli/orange flower oil is reported to be devoid of any irritating properties following at least 20 patch tests with no dermatitis development.

snakeroot oil (Asarum canadensis) Aristolochiaceae
[oral toxicity at 4.48g/kg]
The essential oil of snakeroot is obtained by steam distillation of the macerated dried rhizomes after their trituration with water. It is used only to a limited extent in perfumery.

Composition: 36-46% methyl eugenol, 28-40% linalyl acetate, 5-15% linalool, 2% bornyl acetate, 1.36% geranyl acetate, 1.7% elemicin, 1-1.7% myrcene, 1-1.5% a-pinene, 1-1.35% b-pinene, 1.5% a-terpineol, 1.4% terpinen-4-ol, 1.4% junenol, 1.3% geraniol, 0.9% trans-isoelemicin, 0.8% aristolene, 0.6% eugenol, 0.4% 1,8-cineole, 0.3% methyl thymol and 0.28% sedanolide. [Perfumer & Flavourist (1986) Vol.11 No.1 pgs.47-8]

The following essential oils were tested at a slightly higher concentration than the others in this section which were tested at 4%.

Spanish marjoram oil (Thymus mastichiana) Labiatae - 6%

Both Spanish marjoram (Thymus mastichiana) and Spanish oregano (Thymus capitatus) are species of thyme. Spanish marjoram oil is used mainly in the manufacture of fragrances for both soaps and shampoos. Additionally, there is also some use in the food industry as flavourings. Unlike the garden thyme (Thymus vulgaris) the essential oil of Spanish marjoram contains 1,8-cineole as its principal constituent with linalool and others.
[Perfumer & Flavourist (1980) Vol.5 No.3 pgs.65-7]

lavandin oil (Lavandula hybrida) Labiatae - 5%

Lavandin is a hybrid plant crossed between true lavender and spike lavender. It is cultivated as three main varieties: Abrialis, Super and Grosso. Their composition varies slightly, the Grosso variety having the lowest level of trans-ocimene & 3-octanone and the highest level of terpinen-4-ol, the Super variety having the highest level of linalyl acetate, and the Abralis variety having the highest level of linalool. [Perfumer & Flavourist (1979) Vol.4 No.4 pgs.54]

cypress oil (Cupressus sempervirens) Cupressaceae - 5%

Cypress oil is obtained by steam distillation of the cones from the cypress tree. The essential oil is produced in southern France, Spain and occasionally in other Mediterranean countries including Algeria. The main variable in the commercial oil is a lower level of cedrol at about 5% instead of 20% and almost twice the levels of a-pinene and d-3-carene.
[Perfumer & Flavourist (1976) Vol.1 No.6 pgs.32]

cabreuva oil (Murocarpus frondosus & fastigiatus) Leguminosae - 6%

The essential oil of cabreuva is steam distilled from the aromatic heartwood. In perfumery, it is considered to be an excellent fixative.

Composition: >65% nerolidol, 2.5% farnesol, bisabolol, a-terpineol, and traces of tetrahydro-delta-p-toluic aldehyde and p-methyl acetophenone.

The essential oil of cabreuva seeds contains 26% cadinol.
[Perfumer & Flavourist (1983) Vol.8 No.1 pgs.61-2]

Cabreuva oil is not yet included in the approved lists of both the U.S. Food and Drug Administration and the Council of Europe.

tested at up to 2% on human volunteers without any irritation or sensitisation reactions

This category includes the two tar oils.

birch tar oil (Betula pendula) Betulaceae [dermal toxicity at >2g/kg]
Birch tar oil has been reported to cause hypersensitivity in the occasional individual.

Birch tar oil is obtained by destructive distillation of the wood and bark of the silver birch. It is thick and brownish-black in colour with an agreeable penetrating odour. Birch tar oil has been used in the treatment of eczema, psoriasis and other chronic skin diseases as a cream or ointment containing up to 8%. [Martindale's Extra-Pharmacopoeia 28th ed. 1982]

cade tar oil (Juniperus oxycedrus) Cupressaceae
Cade tar oil has been reported to be a slight local allergen.

Cade tar oil is obtained by destructive distillation of the branches and wood of the cade juniper tree. It is oily and dark reddish-brown, nearly black in colour with an empyreumatic (burnt) odour and an acrid taste. Cade tar oil has been used as an ointment and shampoo in the treatment of psoriasis and as an ointment for the treatment of eczema. It has been incorporated in medicated soaps and has also been used for seborrhoea.
[Martindale's Extra-Pharmacopoeia 28th ed. 1982]

The tar oils are quite strong and are not always suitable for individuals with sensitive skin. The recommendation for topical application is usually to start with as low as 0.25% and gradually increase the concentration according to tolerance; for most people, they are quite safe at up to 2%. The tar oils are sometimes administered orally for respiratory problems, however, they are both irritating to the mucous membrane and the oral toxicity signs of cade tar oil (in rats) includes gastrointestinal irritation and depression.

tested at up to 1% on human volunteers without any irritation or sensitisation reactions

ambrette seed oil (Hibiscus ablemoschus) Malvaceae
The essential oil of ambrette is steam distilled from the seeds and the crude distillate is further refined. The plant is an evergreen shrub, about 1.2 metres in height, cultivated in Egypt and India. Ambrette seed oil contains a macrocyclic lactone, 7-hexadecen-16-olide (ambrettolide) at about 5% that is responsible for its musky fragrance and another macrocyclic lactone, 5-tetradecen-14-olide at about 0.5%, displaying a powerful floral-musky fragrance that is stronger but less tenacious. The oil of plants from China contains up to 15% of ambrettolide.

Composition: 39% farnesol E E, 3.3% farnesol Z E, 35.4% farnesyl acetate E E, 5.8% farnesyl acetate Z E, 3.4% cyclo-dedecene, 1.2% nerolidol, 0.9% trans-jasmone, 0.78% cis-jasmone and 0.2% docecyl acetate, plus the macrocyclic lactones.
[Perfumer & Flavourist (1978) Vol.3 No.4 pgs.54 & (1990) Vol.16 No.5 pgs.80-1]

angelica seed oil (Angelica archangelica) Umbelliferae
Angelica seed oil does not possess the phototoxic potential of angelica root oil.

juniper oil, Phoenician (Juniperus phoenicia) Cupressaceae
Unlike savin oil obtained from Juniperus sabina which is extremely toxic, Phoenician juniper oil obtained from Juniperus phoenicia is safe to use at the recommended concentrations In 1982 the RIFM published specification guidelines for Phoenician juniper oil to avoid confusion with savin oil, which is recommended not to be used as a fragrance by the IFRA.

fir needle oil, Siberian (Abies sibirica) Pinaceae
[dermal toxicity at >3g/kg] *[not tested for phototoxicity]*
Tested at 2.5% on 25 volunteers for 48 hours under close patch, fir needle oil, Siberian produced a mild irritation reaction but did not produce any sensitisation reactions.

spruce oil (Picea mariana & glauca) Pinaceae
The North American production of spruce oil is limited to 4000 - 5000 lbs annually from the provinces of Ontario and Quebec in Canada. The commercial oil is often a mixture of oils from different types of conifer trees. True spruce oil can only be determined by sophisticated analysis. [Perfumer & Flavourist (1979) Vol.3 No.6 pgs.30]

Spruce balsam tested at 20% in 1247 patients for 48 hours produced 62 sensitisation reactions. However spruce oil tested at 1% on 40 volunteers and retested again on 24 volunteers did not produce any sensitisation reactions in either group.

Group I Grade 2 -
low toxicity & hazard with higher dermal toxicity

This group of essential oils exhibits a dermal toxicity value at twice that of their oral toxicity value. The oral toxicity is similar to the Grade 1 essential oils at a theoretical toxic dose of 350 ml for a 70 kg adult, but the dermal toxicity is at 175 ml. They are classified in a separate category to distinguish the higher dermal toxicity. However, safety application in aromatherapy for the Grade 2 essential oils is comparable to that for the Grade 1 essential oils.

geranium oil, Algerian (Pelargonium graveolens) Geraniaceae - 10%
geranium oil, Moroccan (Pelargonium graveolens) Geraniaceae - 10%
geranium oil, Bourbon (Pelargonium graveolens) Geraniaceae - 10%

The Unites States NIOSH concurs with the RIFM on the oral toxicity value of geranium oil. Geraniums are native to South Africa. Contact with Bourbon geranium leaves has been reported to produce vesicular dermatitis and cosmetics containing Bourbon geranium oil may produce dermatitis in hypersensitive individuals. Algerian geranium oil tested at 20% on healthy subjects and at 2% on dermatosis patients did not produce any irritation reactions.

rose oil, Bulgarian (Rosa damascena) Rosaceae - 2%
rose oil, Turkish (Rosa damascena) Rosaceae - 2%
rose oil, Moroccan (Rosa centifolia) Rosaceae - 2%

Essential oil of rose obtained by distillation is called 'attar' or 'otto'. The best rose attar comes from Bulgaria, where rose cultivation for perfumery was established during the period of the Turkish Ottoman Empire of which it was a province. Modern rose cultivation in both Bulgaria and Turkey uses the damask rose (Rosa damascena). The other important centre of rose cultivation is in the Grasse region of southern France where the cabbage rose (Rosa centifolia) is cultivated instead. Moroccan rose cultivation follows the French and uses the cabbage rose. Rose attars are very sensitive to growing conditions and quality very much depends on vintage.

sage oil, clary French (Salvia sclarea) Labiatae - 8%
sage oil, clary Russian (Salvia sclarea) Labiatae *[not tested for toxicity]* - 8%

Clary sage oil from Russia was not tested by the RIFM for oral or dermal toxicity. They are tentatively assumed to be similar to that of clary sage oil from France. Cases of dermatitis caused by clary sage oil have been reported. However, positive patch tests have been obtained only from the mucous membranes but not from the skin.

lavender oil, spike/aspic (Lavandula latifolia) Labiatae - 8%

[not tested for phototoxicity] [oral toxicity at 3.8g/kg]
Spike lavender has become especially established in Spain where it is an important essential oil crop. Lavender, lavandin and spike lavender oils can be distinguished by determining their chemical composition. Spike lavender oil has the lowest ester content of the three lavender oils, being rich in cineole at 35% instead and is dermally twice as toxic as both lavender and lavandin oils. [Perfumer & Flavourist (1980) Vol.5 No.1 pgs.58]

(Eucalyptus citriodora) oil. Myrtaceae - 10%

The chemical composition of the different Eucalyptus oils differs widely. Eucalyptus citriodora oil is second in importance only to Eucalyptus globulus oil. The main constituent of E. citriodora oil is citronellal at over 70% instead of cineole as in E. globulus oil.

Group I Grade 3 - expressed citrus essential oils

The citrus essential oils are distinctive as the only major group extracted by direct expression without distillation. They all have low irritation and sensitisation potential with low-level toxicity. The oral and dermal toxicity values of all the citrus oils exceed the theoretical toxic dose of 350 ml for a 70 kg adult. They have been tested from 5% for tangerine oil to 30% for bergamot oil without producing any irritation or sensitisation reactions. Grapefruit, sweet orange and lemon were retested at 100% for 24 hours with similar negative results. Except for hypersensitive individuals, the citrus oils are safe, used at recommended aromatherapy doses.

The most significant hazard of the citrus oils is their phototoxicity. Without being distilled, the expressed oils contain a proportion of non-volatile components which include the furocoumarins that are responsible for the phototoxic effects.

citrus essential oils (expressed)	furocoumarin average content *	phototoxicity at 100%	conc. when not phototoxic *
bergamot oil (Citrus bergamia)	0.44%	severe	1 - 2%
lime oil (Citrus aurantifolia)	0.25%	strong	2 - 3.5%
bitter orange oil (Citrus aurantium)	0.072%	moderate	3.5 - 7%
lemon oil (Citrus limon)	0.0032%	weak	5 - 10%
grapefruit oil (Citrus paradisi)	0.0012%	weak	10 - 20 %
sweet orange oil (Citrus sinensis)	0.00005%	mild	no limit
tangerine oil (Citrus reticulata)	0.00005%	mild	no limit
mandarin oil (Citrus nobilis)	trace	mild	no limit
tangelo oil (C. reticulata x paradisi)	unknown	mild	no limit

[tangelo is a hybrid of tangerine and grapefruit]

The phototoxic potential of expressed citrus oils is neutralised when the furocoumarin content is reduced to 0.0075% and below. Recommended safe levels for the citrus oils are calculated according to their natural furocoumarin content. The lower limit values are for using each citrus oil on its own; when used in a blend with other non-phototoxic essential oils, the quenching effect allows for a higher safe level of use for the citrus oils.

* The upper limit values are recommendations by the International Fragrance Association (IFRA) for use of the citrus oils in compounds. [The IFRA's guidelines and recommendations on citrus oil were published in Perfumer & Flavourist (1980) Vol.5 No.1 pgs.1-17 and the IFRA's amendments to the guidelines were published in Perfumer & Flavourist (1992) Vol.17 No.6 pgs.66-8]

* [Information on the respective levels of phototoxic furocoumarins in the citrus oils is published as a special feature in the 'Progress in Essential Oils' section of Perfumer & Flavourist (1982) Vol.7 No.3 pgs.57-65]

Group I Grade 4 - oral toxicity at over 3.5g/kg to under 4.5g/kg

bois de rose oil (Aniba rosaedora) Lauraceae [oral toxicity at 4.3g/kg] -12%

The bois de rose tree also known as Brazilian rosewood tree is of slow growth and propagation is difficult. Seasonal variations may cause the linalool content to vary from 36 - 94%. The essential oil is steam distilled from the water-soaked, chipped wood.

Composition: 82-90% linalool, 1.5% cis-linalool oxide, 1.3% trans-linalool oxide, 1% 1,8-cineole, 0.6% b-phellandrene, 0.6% limonene, 0.5% b-pinene, 0.15% a-pinene, (Total monoterpene content: 2 - 2.4%) 3.54% a-terpineol, 0.4% terpinen-4-ol, 0.14% geranyl acetate, 0.03% caryophyllene. (Total sesquiterpene content: 2 - 4.4%).
[Perfumer & Flavourist (1984) Vol.9 No.5 pgs.87-8]

Bois de rose oil did not produce any irritation or sensitisation reactions when tested at 100% under occlusion on a subject with perfume dermatitis.

coriander oil (Coriandrum sativum) Umbelliferae - 6%

[oral toxicity at 4.13g/kg] *[not tested for phototoxicity]*
The United States NIOSH concurs with the RIFM on the oral toxicity value of coriander oil.
The composition of coriander oil is similar to that of bois de rose oil, both containing a high level of linalool. Coriander oil contains the d- isomer of linalool. Both oils also exhibit comparable oral toxicity, with coriander oil being marginally more toxic than bois de rose oil.

dill herb oil (Anethum graveolens) Umbelliferae [oral toxicity at 4.0g/kg]- 4%

The dill plant is reported to be a photosensitising agent. However, the RIFM test results showed dill herb oil to be non-photosensitising.

parsley seed oil (Petroselinum sativum) Umbelliferae -2%

[oral toxicity at 3.96g/kg]
The United States NIOSH concurs with the RIFM on the oral toxicity value of parsley seed oil.
The parsley plant is toxic to chickens, a dose of 17.8g/kg caused diarrhoea, convulsions, paralysis and death. A single dose of 10ml/kg of parsley seed extract in mice caused anuria, drowsiness, dyspnoea and hyperaemia of the viscera with death after 24-60 hours. However no toxic effects were observed in dogs at doses as high as 60g/kg.

cajeput oil (Melaleuca leucodendron) Myrtaceae [oral toxicity at 3.9g/kg] 4%

The United States NIOSH concurs with the RIFM on the oral toxicity value of cajeput oil.
Cajeput oil is more toxic than camphor oil, white, but comparable to laurel leaf oil.

laurel leaf oil (Laurus nobilis) Lauraceae [oral toxicity at 3.95g/kg] - 2%

Laurel leaf oil applied at 2 - 10% has been shown in tests not to produce any irritation or sensitisation reactions in healthy volunteers. However, contact allergy to the oil as topical medicament is common in some European countries, causing hyperaemia and severe inflammation. The allergen in laurel leaf oil is an unsaturated ketone. (It will also produce cross-sensitisation reactions in individuals sensitised to costus oil). **Reduce to 0.1% for hypersensitive individuals.**

fennel seed oil, sweet (Foeniculum vulgare) Umbelliferae - 4%
[oral toxicity at 3.8g/kg]
The oral toxicity of fennel seed oil, sweet, was determined by the Unites States NIOSH to be 3.12g/kg, rating it slightly more toxic than was determined by the RIFM. According to the RIFM test results, fennel seed oil, sweet, appear to be more toxic than fennel seed oil, bitter.

mace oil (Myristica fragrans) Myristicaceae [oral toxicity at 3.64g/kg] - 8%

Mace is the aril that surrounds the nutmeg which is the seed of the nutmeg fruit. Mace oil is chemically similar to nutmeg oil but is slightly less toxic. Safety application is comparable for both oils.

As with nutmeg oil, large doses of mace oil may cause epileptiform convulsions. Toxic symptoms can be caused by a teaspoonful of mace powder. A youth who drank a suspension of powdered mace became hot, weak and dizzy after 4 - 5 hours. Following routine treatment for septic shock, the patient complained only about heaviness in the abdomen. Recovery was rapid and complete. [N Y St J Med (1965) 65/2270]

flouve oil (Anthoxanthum odoratum) Graminae [oral toxicity at 4.1g/kg] - 4%

Flouve is a spring grass widely distributed throughout Eurasia. It has little food value but has been used as fodder. The stems contain large quantities of coumarin which may be recognised by chewing the stalk. Coumarin has the characteristic scent of newly mown hay. Extracts of the juice of the whole grass but not of the pollen were reported to produce a positive reaction in a subject with summer asthma.

Flouve oil is not yet included in the approved lists of both the U.S. Food and Drug Administration and the Council of Europe.

Group I Grade 5 - oral toxicity at over 2.5g/kg to under 3.5g/kg

elemi oil (Canarium commune) Burseraceae [oral toxicity at 3.4g/kg] - 4%
Elemi oil is obtained by the distillation of the resinous exudate of the Manila elemi tree that is native to the Philippines.

Composition: 2.4% myrcene, 15% a-phellandrene, 54% limonene, 2.5% 1,8-cineole, 1.5% p-cymene, 15% elemol and 3.5% elemicin. [Perfumer & Flavourist (1980) Vol.5 No.1 pgs.58]

lovage oil (Levisticum officinale) Umbelliferae [oral toxicity at 3.4g/kg] - 2%
Lovage is a vigorous plant native to southern Europe. The essential oil is steam distilled from the roots, having an aroma reminiscent of celery but is somewhat sweeter and heavier. A case of sensitivity to lovage oil has been reported. However, the RIFM test results showed lovage oil to be non-sensitising.

parsley herb oil (Petroselinum sativum) Umbelliferae - 2%
[oral toxicity at 3.3g/kg]
Parsley herb oil obtained from the whole plant is very similar to parsley leaf oil, however they both differ slightly from parsley seed oil. According to the RIFM test results, parsley herb oil appears to be slightly more toxic than parsley seed oil.

ho leaf oil (Cinnamomum camphora) Lauraceae - 10%
[oral toxicity at 3.27g/kg] *[not tested for phototoxicity]*
The United States NIOSH concurs with the RIFM on the oral toxicity value of ho leaf oil.
Ho leaf oil is obtained by steam distillation of the leaves of the linaloola chemotype camphor tree from Taiwan, known locally as 'ho shu'. Recently more ho leaf oil production has been carried out in China with Japan providing a much smaller secondary source. Ho leaf oil contains up to 80% of linalool. [Perfumer & Flavourist (1979) Vol.4 No.4 pgs.53]

pine oil, yarmor (Pinus palustris) Pinaceae [oral toxicity at 3.2gkg] - 12%
A 31 year old woman induced an abortion by instilling into her uterus about 75 to 150 ml of a 1 in 3 mixture of yarmor pine oil and soap in water. She developed acute renal failure within 24 hours, with vomiting and widely distributed pain. The uraemia slowly cleared but anaemia, present when the patient was admitted to hospital, persisted for nearly 6 months. A peripheral neuropathy which occurred at 4 weeks after abortion gradually subsided. Focal fibrosis and tubular atrophy were present 6 weeks after admission to hospital. [J Am med Ass (1968) 203/146]

Recommended limit of use at 2%.

clove bud oil (Eugenia caryophyllata) Myrtaceae [oral toxicity at 2.7g/kg] 5%
clove stem oil (Eugenia caryophyllata) Myrtaceae [oral toxicity at 2.9g/kg]

Clove bud and stem oils are used as a domestic remedy for toothache, a plug of cotton wool soaked in the oil being inserted in the cavity of the carious tooth. Repeated application may damage the gingival (gum) tissue. Clove bud oil is slightly less toxic than clove stem oil, however clove leaf oil seems to be significantly more toxic than both clove bud and stem oils.

Daily oral doses at 0.35 - 0.7g/kg for 8 weeks were well tolerated in rats. Higher doses caused inactivity and weight loss. Tested at 20% in an ointment on 25 volunteers, clove bud and stem oils produced 2 irritation reactions. They did not produce any irritation reactions when retested at 2% on healthy subjects and at 0.1% on patients with dermatosis.

cinnamon leaf oil (Cinnamomum zeylanicum) Lauraceae - 10%
[oral toxicity at 2.65g/kg]
Cinnamon leaf oil and the three clove oils all contain a high content of eugenol at up to 80%. According to the RIFM test results, cinnamon leaf oil appeared to be similar to clove bud oil in toxicity. The United States NIOSH determined the oral toxicity values of cinnamon leaf and clove bud at 4.16g/kg and 3.72g/kg respectively, rating them to be less toxic than by the RIFM.

nutmeg oil (Myristica fragrans) Myristicaceae [oral toxicity at 2.62g/kg] - 2%
The United States NIOSH concurs with the RIFM on the oral toxicity value of nutmeg oil.
Lethal doses of nutmeg oil cause fatty degeneration of the liver and central nervous system paralysis in animals. The liver changes have been attributable to the myristicin content of nutmeg oil. Several cases of intoxication have been reported. Taken in large doses, nutmeg oil may cause nausea and vomiting, flushing or sometimes shivering, dry mouth, tachycardia, disorientation, stupor or stimulation of the central nervous system possibly with epileptiform convulsions, miosis sometimes followed by mydriasis, and euphoria and hallucinations.
[Martindale's Extra-Pharmacopoeia 28th ed. 1982]

In 1960, 2 Swedish girls ingesting 15 - 25g of powdered nutmeg, experienced impaired visual perception, sleeping continuously for 40 hours and waking up in a euphoric state; the intoxication is dose dependent and their symptoms lasted for 10 days.

star anise oil (Illicium verum) Illiciaceae [oral toxicity at 2.6g/kg] - 4%
Both star anise and aniseed oils contain a high content of trans-antheole (85%). According to the RIFM test results, star anise oil appeared to be slightly less toxic than aniseed oil.

sage oil, Dalmation (Salvia officinalis) Labiatae [oral toxicity at 2.6g/kg] - 8%
The United States NIOSH concurs with the RIFM on the oral toxicity value of D. sage oil.
Retested at 100% for 24 hours on 20 volunteers. D. sage oil produced 1 irritation reaction.

Group I Grade 6 - oral toxicity at over 1.5g/kg to under 2.5g/kg

Peru balsam oil (Myroxylon pereirae) Leguminosae - 8%
[oral toxicity at 2.36g/kg]
The United States NIOSH concurs with the RIFM on the oral toxicity value of Peru balsam oil. Peru balsam oil extracted by distillation is free from allergens found in the crude balsam.

anise oil (Pimpinella anisum) Umbelliferae [oral toxicity at 2.25g/kg] - 2%
The anise plant was found to contain a volatile insecticidal agent identified as the trans-anethole which could kill houseflies at 75 microgrammes.

Composition: 1% methyl chavicol, 2.3% cis-anethole, 85% trans-antheole, 0.5% safrole, 1% anisaldehyde and 1% acetoanisole. [Perfumer & Flavourist (1983) Vol.8 No.3 pgs.65-6]

Anise oil is not a primary irritant to human skin but several cases of sensitisation have been reported causing dermatitis consisting of erythema, desquamation and vesiculation. **Reduce to 0.1% for hypersensitive individuals.**

marjoram oil (Origanum marjoranum) Labiatae - 6%
[oral toxicity at 2.24g/kg] *[not tested for phototoxicity]*
Marjoram oil occurs in two forms: one predominant in terpinen-4-ol and the other predominant in cis-thujanol-4 (cis-sabinene hydrate). These compounds are biogenetically related and the chemical composition of various marjoram oils are quantitative variations on a central biosynthetic theme. [Perfumer & Flavourist (1976) Vol.1 No.2 pgs.18]

Composition: 2-5.4% trans-ocimene & g-terpinene, 2-3.4% p-cymene, 0.5-1% terpinelene, 1-3.6% trans-thujanol-4, 1.5% linalool, 3.4-11.4% cis-thujanol-4, 3.2% linalyl acetate, 20-25% terpinen-4-ol, 3.5% terpinen-4-yl acetate, 2.4% caryophyllene, 5% a-terpineol, 1% carvone, 11-17% thymol and 19-25% carvacrol. [Perfumer & Flavourist (1981) Vol.6 No.5 pgs.28-32]

tarragon oil (Artemisia dracunculus) Compositae [oral toxicity at 1.9g/kg] 4%
Tarragon is cultivated in two forms: the French is a fine aromatic sterile plant and the Russian is a scrubbier, weakly aromatic, seed producing perennial. Tarragon or estragon oil is distilled from the leaves, mainly produced in France and used in perfumery particularly in France and Italy, and also in food flavouring. [Perfumer & Flavourist (1988) Vol.13 No.1 pgs.49-50]

Composition: 2.5-4% limonene, 6.6-9.3% cis-ocimene, 7.5-10.5% trans-ocimene & g-terpinene, and 60-80% methyl chavicol (estragole).
[Perfumer & Flavourist (1990) Vol.15 No.2 pgs.75-6]

tea tree oil (Melaleuca alternifolia) Myrtaceae [oral toxicity at 1.9g/kg] - 1%

Tea tree is a tree native to Australia, that is related to the cajeput tree of Malaysia. The essential oil is distilled from the leaves that were formerly used for brewing by the early settlers in Australia as a substitute for tea (Camellia chinensis).

Composition: 2.8% a-pinene, 29.4% terpinen-4-ol, 16.5% 1,8-cineole, 11.5% g-terpinene, 11.4% p-cymene, 2.36% terpinolene, 3.6% a-terpineol, 1% viridiflorene and 1.4% a-cadinene.
[Perfumer & Flavourist (1978) Vol.3 No.5 pgs.41]

bay oil (Pimenta racemosa) Myrtaceae - 10%

[oral toxicity at 1.8g/kg] *[not tested for phototoxicity]*
The essential oil of bay is obtained by steam distillation of the leaves. A major portion of the world's supply comes from the island of Dominica with a second source from Puerto Rico.

Composition: 0.1-1% a-pinene, 5.7-14% myrcene, 1.4-2.2% limonene, 0.2-26% 1,8-cineole, 1.7-2% linalool, 20-56% eugenol, 1% 3-octanone, 1-4.2% 1-octen-3-ol and 21.6% chavicol.
[Perfumer & Flavourist (1977) Vol.2 No.6 pgs.36]

sweet birch oil (Betula lenta) Betulaceae [oral toxicity at 1.7g/kg] - 4%

Sweet birch oil is chemically similar to wintergreen oil, both containing up to 99% of methyl salicylate. It is pale yellow in colour with the characteristic odour of methyl salicylate.

A 6 year old boy sensitive to aspirin, developed generalised pustular psoriasis consequent to walking in the woodland of eastern Pennsylvania in April, inhaling pollen and chewing twigs of sweet birch and the leaves of wintergreen, both of which contained methyl salicylate.
[J Am med Ass (1964) 189/985]

myrrh oil (Commiphora myrrha) Burseraceae [oral toxicity at 1.65g/kg] - 8%

The myrrh tree is fairly small, almost shrub-like in appearance, commonly found in small thickets. It is a thorny tree with a gnarled trunk and ash-grey coloured branches. Commiphora species can be found in Somalia, Eritrea, Ethiopia, Yemen and Saudi Arabia, yielding an oleo-gum-resin. Myrrh oil is used in perfumery for fragrances with heavy floral, woody, balsamic, pine forest and mossy notes.

Composition: 1.5% p-cymene, 1.9% cis-ocimene, 1.27% trans-ocimene, 28.8% d-elemene, 10% copaene, 5% bourbonene, 6.2% b-elemene, 5% bergamotene, with 1.93% methylfuran, 5.68% methyl isobutyl ketone, 2.23% 3-methyl-2-butenal, 2.84% xylenes, 1.44% furfural, 1.18% 2-methyl-5-isopropylfuran, 1% 4,4—dimethyl-2-butenolide, 1.66% 5-methylfurfural and 4.63% 2-methyl-5-isopropenylfuran. [Perfumer & Flavourist (1983) Vol.8 No.5 pgs.22-5]

Group I Grade 7 - oral toxicity at over 0.5g/kg to under 1.5g/kg

basil oil (Ocimum basilicum) Labiatae [oral toxicity at 1.4g/kg] - 4%

Two main types of basil oil are commercially available: Reunion basil oil containing a high content of methyl chavicol (estragole) and European basil oil containing approximately equal proportions of methyl chavicol and linalool. A third type of basil oil from India and Africa is also available containing a high content of methyl cinnamate.
[Perfumer & Flavourist (1978) Vol.3 No.5 pgs.36-8]

Composition of **basil oil from Comoro Island**: 85.7% methyl chavicol, 1.2% linalool, 2.6% limonene, 1.2% fenchyl alcohol and 0.8% a-terpineol.
Composition of **basil oil from France**: 40.7% linalool, 23.8% methyl chavicol, 2% limonene, 6.7% fenchyl alcohol and 2% a-terpineol. [Perfumer & Flavourist (1980) Vol.4 No.6 pgs.31]

The sample tested by the RIFM was the European basil oil containing up to 55% of methyl chavicol and 35% linalool.

Another species of basil, O. gratissimum from Africa, produces an essential oil that contains 60-80% eugenol. This species of basil is widely grown in Russia and is also grown in India.
[Perfumer & Flavourist (1987) Vol.12 No.5 pgs.80]

hyssop oil (Hyssopus officinalis) Labiatae [oral toxicity at 1.4g/kg] - 4%

Hyssop oil is quite uncommon, it is sometimes used for seasoning in Europe but its greatest use is in flavouring preparations for alcoholic beverages.

Composition: 32.6% isopinocamphone, 12.2% pinocamphone, 23% b-pinene, 4.8% caryophyllene, 2.4% limonene, 2.2% spathulenol, 2% germacrene D & d-cadinene, 1.8% myrcene, 1.7% b-elemol, 1.4% a-pinene, 1.3% estragole and 1% mertenol & a-humelene.
[Perfumer & Flavourist (1977) Vol.2 No.2 pgs.30]

Certain essential oils containing high levels of ketones have been incriminated in convulsive poisonings in France. The presence of the 2 ketones, pinocamphone and isopinocamphone in hyssop oil accounted for its toxicity which caused epileptic crises and cortical and muscular manifestations (in rats). [Perfumer & Flavourist (1984) Vol.9 No.3 pgs.38]

cornmint oil (Mentha arvensis) Labiatae [oral toxicity at 1.24g/kg] - 8%

In a study evaluating the comparative action of skin-penetrating agents, cornmint oil increased deep penetration (of Rhodamine B) in the epidermis and dermis of guineapig skin while peppermint oil only caused a slight increase in penetration.

Composition: 3.4-14.8% menthone, 1.9-4.8% isomenthone, 1-2.5% methyl acetate, 0.8-1.5% neomenthol, 65-80% menthol, 0.2-1.6% piperitone. [Perfumer & Flavourist (1981) Vol.6 No.4 pgs.73]

The essential oil of cornmint is often dementholised by freeze crystallisation, removing up to 48% of pure menthol crystals leaving 32-40% of menthol in the oil.
[Perfumer & Flavourist (1983) Vol.8 No.2 pgs.61-3]

Cornmint oil produced moderate cytotoxic effects which could not be attributed to its content of menthol at up to 85% and related methyl compounds.

tansy oil (Tanacetum vulgare) Compositae [oral toxicity at 1.15g/kg] - 4%

Tansy oil like several others from the Compositae family occurs as many chemotypes. The major constituent is usually thujone, however tansy oils have also been found with the following compounds as a major constituent: isothujone, camphone, artemisone, isopinocamphone, umbellulone, g-terpinene, borneol, bornyl acetate, cis-chrysanthenyl acetate, piperitone and its sesquiterpene derivative. [Perfumer & Flavourist (1976) Vol.1 No.1 pgs.4]

The average content of both a- and b- thujones combined in tansy oil is about 50%. Essential oils containing large amounts of thujone are poisonous causing convulsions and epileptic-like attacks. The oral toxicity values (in rats) of thujone and tansy oil are 0.3g/kg and 1.15g/kg respectively. Thujone is three and a half times more toxic. Signs of tansy oil poisoning due to thujone include vomiting, gastro-enteritis, flushing, cramps, loss of consciousness, rapid breathing, irregular heart beat, rigid pupils, uterine bleeding and hepatitis. Death results from circulatory and respiratory arrest and organ degeneration.

When administered in test animals in increasing amounts, doses twice as large as the toxic dose could be tolerated.

wormwood oil (Artemisia absinthum) Compositae - 2%

[oral toxicity at 0.96g/kg]
Wormwood is a species of the genus Artemisia. The essential oil is produced in Spain, Italy, Germany and Russia and is of only minor importance, used in limited quantities in fragrance compounding and in some external analgesics. [Perfumer & Flavourist (1981) Vol.6 No.2 pgs.63]

Composition: 2.7% sabinene, 1% myrcene, 2.76% a-thujone, 46.44% b-thujone, 3.2% trans-sabinol, 27.78% trans-sabinyl acetate & linalyl acetate and 1.4% geranyl propionate.
[Perfumer & Flavourist (1992) Vol.17 No.2 pgs.39-44]

Another species of Artemisia, A. annua (annual wormwood) is also used to produce an essential oil in Yugoslavia and Bulgaria, having a ketone content of 22-34%.
[Perfumer & Flavourist (1977) Vol.2 No.2 pgs.32]

Group I Grade 8 - high oral toxicity

thuja leaf oil (Thuja occidentalis) Cupressaceae
[oral toxicity at 0.83g/kg & dermal toxicity at 4.1g/kg]
The United States NIOSH concurs with the RIFM on the oral toxicity value of thuja leaf oil.

Thuja leaf oil is obtained by steam distillation of the leaves and twigs of the thuja tree obtained from the wild state as the tree is not cultivated. Thuja is native to the Great Lakes-St. Lawrence region of Canada, distributed from Winnepeg in the west to Nova Scotia in the east and as far north as James Bay. In the United States, it is found in the northern New England states, upper New York state and upper Michigan. The traditional areas of thuja leaf oil production are in New York and Vermont in the U.S. and eastern Quebec and southeastern Ontario in Canada. Production has always been a small local industry totalling not more than 60, 000 lbs annually.
[Perfumer & Flavourist (1979) Vol.3 No.6 pgs.28-9]

Used since the mid-19th century in the manufacture of externally applied patent medicines, thuja leaf oil is also used for room deodorants and fragrances where a herbal note is wanted.

Composition: 1.3% a-pinene, 1.2% camphene, 1.8% d-sabinene, 1% d-limonene, 1.4% p-cymene, 14% l-fenchone, 60% a-thujone, 9.5% b-thujone, 2% camphone, 1.2% terpinen-4-ol and 2.3% bornyl acetate. [Perfumer & Flavourist (1979) Vol.4 No.1 pgs.48]

armoise oil (Artemisia vulgaris) Compositae
[oral toxicity at 0.37g/kg & dermal toxicity at >5g/kg]
The armoise plant is a native of Europe belonging to the abrotanum section of the large and complex genus, Artemisia. An essential oil can be obtained from this plant with a thuja leaf-like odour due to the constituent, thujone occurring in both essential oils.

A north African species belonging to the seriphidium section of Artemisia, A. herba-alba is also used for producing an essential oil. This plant is not cultivated but collected from the wild and distilled in Morocco. Artemisia herba-alba occurs as 7 recognised chemotypes.

Composition of **European armoise oil**: 1.4% a-thujene, 1.3% a-pinene, 1.44% camphene, 16% sabinene, 1.4% b-pinene, 14% myrcene, 9.75% 1,8-cineole, 1.6% g-terpinene, 1% trans-sabinene hydrate, 1.8% camphone, 2.2% vulgarol, 6% cubenene & aromadendrene, 2% terpinen-4-ol, 3.4% guaiene and 1.5% g-elemene.

Composition of **Moroccan armoise oil (a-thujone chemotype)**: 2.6% camphene, 2% 1,8-cineole, 36-82% a-thujone, 6-16% b-thujone, 1.6% chrysanthenone and 15% camphone.
Composition of **Moroccan armoise oil (b-thujone chemotype)**: 3.5% camphene, 3.8% 1,8-cineole, 0.5-17% a-thujone, 44-94% b-thujone, 2.4% chrysanthenone and 9% camphone.
[Perfumer & Flavourist (1989) Vol.14 No.3 pgs.71-4]

The commercial armoise oil is mostly obtained from A. herba-alba, so the sample tested by the RIFM is probably that of a-thujone chemotype Moroccan armoise oil, having a thujone content similar to that of thuja leaf oil.

pennyroyal oil (Mentha pulegium) Labiatae
[oral toxicity at 0.4g/kg & dermal toxicity at 4.2g/kg]
The United States NIOSH concurs with the RIFM on the oral toxicity value of pennyroyal oil.

Pennyroyal is a European mint and the main country of production is Spain, with smaller production in Portugal, Italy and Yugoslavia. North African pennyroyal oil is distilled in Morocco and Tunisia from the European pennyroyal plant (M. pulegium). Pennyroyal oil has minor importance in fragrance compounding for its herbaceous, slightly minty character.

Composition: 1.5-2% 3-octanol, 0.5-30.8% menthone, 5.2-19.8% isomenthone, 3% neomenthone, 0.3-1.4% neoisomethyl acetate, 0.7-5.8% neoisomenthol and 52-63.5% pulegone.
[Perfumer & Flavourist (1978) Vol.3 No.5 pgs.40]

Pennyroyal oil was formerly used as an emmenagogue. Attempts at abortion using pennyroyal oil have resulted in severe toxic effects with convulsions and death. However, it is recognised that the abortive action is only a secondary effect of the intoxication.
[Perfumer & Flavourist (1979) Vol.4 No.1 pgs.15-17]

The Food Standards Committee recommendation for pennyroyal oil is that it should not be used in foods as a flavouring agent. [Report on flavouring agents (1965) HM Stationery Office, London]

Another plant called American pennyroyal (Hedeoma pulegeoides) of the same family, Labiatae also produces an essential oil very rich in pulegone at 62-82%. This plant is native to eastern North America from Nova Scotia southward and the essential oil is distilled from plants collected from the wild in the midwestern states of Tennessee and North Carolina. However, it is not as important as European pennyroyal oil. [Perfumer & Flavourist (1979) Vol.3 No.6 pgs.33]

Pulegone is the main constituent of both pennyroyal oils from Mentha pulegium and Hedeoma pulegeoides. In comparison to the toxicity of several active constituents of essential oils, pulegone was considered to be less toxic than others. [Deutsche Med Wochenschr (1920) 46/389]

Recommended limit for the essential oils in this category at 2%

Group I Grade 9 - moderate irritation potential

Exert caution in the use of this category of essential oils by maintaining low concentrations at 0.25 - 1% for healthy individuals and **avoid using on hypersensitive individuals.**

Virginian cedarwood oil (Juniperus virginiana) Cupressaceae
Texas cedarwood oil (Juniperus mexicana) Cupressaceae

J. virginiana is a small to medium size tree growing throughout the southeastern U.S. The largest stands occur in middle Tennessee and northern Alabama (where it is often found as the dominant tree) but the major production area for the essential oil is in North Carolina. Annual production is about 450,000 lbs. Early in the 17th century, the wood was used in the manufacture of linen chests due to its agreeable odour and resistance to clothes moths and other insects that eat woollen and cotton fabrics. However, the wood is most important for the manufacture of pencils. The essential oil is obtained by steam distilling the sawdust, chipped logs, old stumps and waste wood as a by-product of the timber industry. It is used in the fragrance industry for sanitation supplies and soap. [Perfumer & Flavourist (1979) Vol.3 No.6 pgs.30]

J. mexicana is a small to medium size tree growing throughout central and western Texas southwards into Mexico and Guatemala at altitudes of 250 - 800 m. The trees are used directly for chips in the production of essential oil at an annual total of 1.2 - 2 million lbs. There is no timber industry for the wood of this tree. The spent fibres after distillation are used as litter absorbent in the animal pet trade. [Perfumer & Flavourist (1979) Vol.3 No.6 pgs.31]

Both the North American species of juniper called 'cedarwood' require some caution in their use. The Texan is reported to be a slight acute or chronic local irritant and allergen; while the Virginian possesses low-level phototoxicity and has been reported to cause pigmentation following topical application. Use of the Virginian, followed by exposure to various types of radiation sometimes causes dermatitis. The chemical composition of both essential oils is very similar, the Texan having a higher content of cedrol than the Virginian.
The recommended limit of use for both oils is 1%.

pine oil, pumilo (Pinus pumilo) Pinaceae

Tested at 12% on 22 volunteers, pumilo pine oil produced 3 irritation reactions without any sensitisation reactions. Safety application regarding the peroxide content is similar to that for Scots pine oil. According to the RIFM test results, pumilo pine oil appears to be a stronger irritant than Scots pine oil. **The recommended limit of use is 1%**

citronella oil (Cymbopogon nardus) Graminae [dermal toxicity at 4.7g/kg]
[not tested for phototoxicity]
Citronella oil is reported to cause hypersensitivity resulting in papulovesicular eczema (rash with both papules and vesicles) of the fingers, hands, forearms and acneform folliculitis (inflammation of the hair follicles). It is considered as a primary irritant and sensitiser in perfumes. However, citronella oil tested at 8% on 25 volunteers for 48 hours by the RIFM did not produce any irritation or sensitisation reactions. **Recommended limit of use at 1%. Avoid using on hypersensitive individuals.**

perilla oil (Perilla frutescens) Labiatae
The perilla plant is much cultivated in East Asia. Naturalised in southeastern Europe particularly in the Ukraine. The leaves are used in Japan as a garnish for shushi.

Perilla oil is reported to cause various dermal effects on the fingers, such as erosion, fissure, desquamation, thickening or bleeding in half the surveyed 152 workers handling perilla plants. Both the leaves and oil produce allergic reactions in workers with dermatitis. However perilla oil tested at 4% on 25 volunteers for 48 hours by the RIFM did not produce any irritation or sensitisation reactions. **Recommended limit of use at 0.5%. Avoid using on patients with dermatitis.**

tagetes oil (Tagetes minuta) Compositae [oral toxicity at 3.7g/kg]
Tagetes is a hardy composite plant native to west central South America. The entire plant is steam distilled to produce a yellowish-red essential oil possessing a pungent but pleasant harsh, wild-herb, semi-rancid note. [Perfumer & Flavourist (1984) Vol.9 No.5 pgs.62]

The tagetes plant is affected in the yield and composition of its essential oil by the availability of nitrogen and phosphorus in the soil. Plants grown in nitrogen-deficient soil produced an oil that is very high in dihydro-tagetone.

Composition: 40.42% (Z)-b-ocimene, 17.74% dihydro-tagetone, 1% (E)-tagetone, 10% (Z)-tagetone, 5.3% (E)-tagetone and 3.5% germacrene D.
[Perfumer & Flavourist (1992) Vol.17 No.5 pgs.131-3]

Following exposure to the fresh leaves and flowers, tagetes was reported to produce primary irritation and severe prolonged allergic contact dermatitis in humans. It did not produce cross-sensitisation reactions in patients previously sensitised to costus absolute. The reported level of use in perfumes is 0.08% with a maximum level of 0.2%. **The IFRA recommendation for tagetes oil is a limit of 0.25% in a compound.** This recommendation is based on test results showing a no-effect level of 0.05% on humans using tagetes absolute. [IFRA Report Oct 86]

Group I Grade 10 - severe phototoxic potential

angelica root oil (Angelica archangelica) Umbelliferae
Composition: 24% a-pinene, 1.3% camphene, 1.25% b-pinene, 10% d-3-carene, 7.6% a-phellandrene & myrcene, 13.2% limonene, 10% b-phellandrene, 1.25% cis-ocimene, 2.68% trans-ocimene, 9.8% p-cymene, 2% a-copaene, 1% b-elemene and 1.2% a-muurolene.
[Perfumer & Flavourist (1977) Vol.1 No.6 pgs.31]

At a daily intake for 8 weeks, the tolerated dose of angelica root oil in rats was 1.5g/kg, but even at a 0.5 - 1g/kg daily dose, it caused a decrease in weight and activity in the tested animals. The lethal oral dose is 11.16g/kg when death is preceded by severe liver and kidney damage. However, test animals surviving for 3 days recovered completely from any liver or kidney damage.

rue oil (Ruta graveolens) Rutaceae
The 3 dominant furocoumarins in rue oil responsible for its phototoxic effect are psoralen, bergapten and xanthotoxin. Dipping the leaves into water at a temperature above 90 degrees C. will remove 1 - 3 times more furocoumarins from the leaf surface than by normal extraction.

Composition: 18% 2-nonanone, 1% 2-decanone, 11% 2-nonyl acetate, 30% 2-undecanone, 1.2% 2-undecyl acetate, 3% 2-butanone, 1.28% psoralen and 7.24% bergapten & xanthotoxin. (Rue oil obtained from plants grown in Malaysia). [Perfumer & Flavourist (1990) Vol.15 No.2 pgs.79]

Rue oil taken internally may produce haemorrhage. Ingestion of large quantities of rue oil causes epigastric pain, nausea, vomiting, confusion, convulsions and death; abortion may result It may harm the mucous membranes and irritate the skin, producing erythema and vesication after frequent dermal contact. **Rue oil is a powerful local irritant.**

The value of rue oil is in flavouring, especially for confectionery and bakery goods. Rue oil is not often used in cosmetics as it has been considered to be harmful to the mucous membranes. The reported powerful irritant effect is presumed to be due to the rapid penetration of rue oil into the skin. [Perfumer & Flavourist (1978) Vol.3 No.2 pgs.48]

Angelica root oil and rue oil tested at 100% were phototoxic on exposure of the skin area to simulated sunlight for 1 hour after application. They still produced distinct reactions at 50%, 25%, 12.5%, 6.25% and 3.12% decreasing to slight reactions at 1.56% and were completely non-phototoxic at 0.78%. **Recommended limit of use for angelica root oil at 1% and rue oil at 0.5%.** The IFRA recommendation for angelica root oil and rue oil is a limit of 3.9% in a compound for application on areas of skin exposed to sunshine. Bath preparations and other products which are washed off the skin are excluded from the limit.
[Angelica root oil - IRFA Report Jun 75/Oct 78] & [Rue oil - IFRA Report Nov 74/Oct 78]

Group I Grade 11 -
moderate to severe sensitisation and phototoxic potential

verbena oil (Lippia citriodora) Verbenaceae

Lippia citriodora is native to South America; Verbena officinalis is the vervain of Europe. Both plants are members of the same Verbenaceae family.

Originally found in Chile and Peru, L. citriodora was introduced into England in 1784 and cultivated in gardens reaching a height of up to 5 metres. The leaves are very fragrant, retaining their odour for years when dried and have been used for brewing as a tea.

Composition: 26% geranial, 12% neral, 6% geraniol, 5.2% nerol, 4.2% limonene, 3% 1,8-cineole, 1.75 heptenone, 1% citronellal, 1% copaene, 3% caryophyllene, 4% neryl acetate, 1.8% germacrene D, 4.8% a-farnescene, 1.8% geranyl acetate, 1% citronellol, 4.5% curcumene, 1.3% nerolidol and 2.5% spathulenol. [Perfumer & Flavourist (1977) Vol.2 No.2 pgs.32]

Verbena oil tested at 12% (using 6 different samples) on 159 volunteers for 48 hours produced 3 irritation reactions.

French verbena oil tested at 100% was phototoxic. Tested at 12% on 25 volunteers, it was not phototoxic but produced 13 sensitisation reactions.

Moroccan verbena oil tested at 100% was phototoxic. Tested at 50% on 25 volunteers, it was not phototoxic but was still irritating. Tested at 12% it produced 4 sensitisation reactions.

Boufarik verbena oil tested at 12% on 30 volunteers did not produce any sensitisation reactions but produced 1 irritation reaction.

The reported maximum concentration of verbena oil in consumer products is 1.2%. **Recommended limit of use is 0.25%.** The IFRA recommendation for verbena oil is that it should not be used as a perfume ingredient. This recommendation is based on the RIFM test results showing the sensitising and phototoxic effects of verbena oil. [IFRA Report Dec 81]

Group I Grade 12 - moderate to severe sensitisation potential

SEVERE SENSITISATION POTENTIAL
costus root oil (Sassurea lappa) Compositae
[oral toxicity at 3.4g/kg & dermal toxicity at >5g/kg]
The United States NIOSH concurs with the RIFM on the oral toxicity value of costus root oil.
elecampane root oil (Inula helenium) Compositae *[not tested for toxicity]*
The RIFM did not test elecampane root oil for oral, dermal or photo-toxicity. They are tentatively assumed to be comparable to that of costus root oil.

Tested at 4% on 25 volunteers, elecampane root oil produced 23 extremely severe sensitisation reactions and costus root oil produced sensitisation reactions in all 25 test volunteers, extremely severely in 8 of them. Tested at 2% on 26 volunteers, costus root oil still produced 16 sensitisation reactions. Both oils produced cross-sensitisation reactions to each other. Anyone sensitised to one oil will be re-sensitised to the other. **The recommended limit of use for both costus root oil and elecampane root oil is 0.1%.** Considering the RIFM test results showing sensitising potential in some samples and absence of sensitising potential in other samples, the IFRA concurs with the recommendation of a limit of 0.1% for costus root oil but tentatively recommends that elecampane root oil should not be used until further studies confirm its safety. The essential oil from both plants contains certain sesquiterpene lactones with an a-methylene butyrolactone structure having a sensitisation potential. [IFRA Report Jun 75]

MODERATE SENSITISATION POTENTIAL
cinnamon bark oil (Cinnamomum zeylanicum) Lauraceae
[oral toxicity at 3.4g/kg & dermal toxicity at 0.69g/kg]
cassia oil (Cinnamomum aromaticum) Lauraceae
[oral toxicity at 2.8g/kg & dermal toxicity at 0.32g/kg]
The United States NIOSH concurs with the RIFM on the oral toxicity value of cassia oil.

In addition to their sensitisation potential, both cassia and cinnamon bark oils also possess low-level phototoxicity which is not considered to be significant when used with other non-phototoxic essential oils, but can enhance the phototoxic potential of other phototoxic essential oils. Tested at 4% and 8% respectively, cassia oil produced 2 and cinnamon bark oil produced 20 sensitisation reactions from 2 groups of 25 test volunteers each. Cassia oil is listed as a sensitiser and after using toothpaste containing cinnamon bark oil, 3 patients developed acute contact sensitivity of the mouth; symptoms subsided within 1 week when the use of the toothpaste ceased. **The IFRA recommendation for using both cassia oil and cinnamon bark oil is a tentative limit of 1%.** These recommendations were based on the RIFM test results showing an absence of sensitisation reactions at these lower concentrations, cassia oil being less sensitising than cinnamon bark oil. [IFRA Report Oct 74/Oct 78/Oct80]

Group I Grade 13 - moderate to high dermal toxicity

MODERATE DERMAL TOXICITY
caraway oil (Carum carvi) Umbelliferae
[oral toxicity at 3.5g/kg & dermal toxicity at 1.7g/kg]
cumin oil (Cuminum cyminum) Umbelliferae
[oral toxicity at 2.5g/kg & dermal toxicity at 3.56g/kg]
The United States NIOSH concurs with the RIFM on the oral toxicity values of both caraway and cumin oils. At 100% caraway oil exhibited only low-level phototoxicity which is not considered to be significant, but cumin oil exhibited distinct phototoxicity. **The IFRA recommendation for cumin oil is to limit the concentration to 2% for application on areas of skin exposed to sunshine**, based on the RIFM test results showing a no-effect level of 5% in phototoxicity tests with human subjects. Bath preparations and other products which are washed off the skin are excluded from this limit. **The recommended limit of use for caraway oil is 4%.**

pimento leaf oil (Pimenta officinalis) Myrtaceae
[oral toxicity at 3.6g/kg & dermal toxicity at 2.82g/kg]
pimento berry oil (Pimenta officinalis) Myrtaceae *[not tested for toxicity]*
The RIFM did not test pimento berry oil for oral or dermal toxicity. They are tentatively assumed to be comparable to that of pimento leaf oil. Pimento trees are grown commercially in Jamaica, but the essential oil obtained from the dried leaves and immature fruits (berries) are distilled in the U.S. Both pimento leaf and berry oils are valued in the flavour and fragrance industries. [Perfumer & Flavourist (1980) Vol.5 No.4 pgs.34]

Composition of pimento leaf oil: 1.4% 1,8-cineole, 7.6% b-caryophyllene, 1% d- & g- cadinene, 2% methyl eugenol and 84% eugenol.
Composition of pimento berry oil: 1.8% a-phellandrene, 4.2% limonene, 3% 1,8-cineole, 1% p-cymene, 1.4% terpinolene, 4% b-caryophyllene, 1% a-humulene, 1.2% b-selinene, 8.6% methyl eugenol and 68% eugenol. [Perfumer & Flavourist (1990) Vol.15 No.1 pgs.63-4]

clove leaf oil (Eugenia caryophyllata) Myrtaceae
[oral toxicity at 1.37g/kg & dermal toxicity at 1.2g/kg]
Of the three types of clove oil commercially available (bud, stem and leaf oils), clove leaf oil is produced in the largest volume but is also the most toxic of the three.

Composition: 95% eugenol, 1% eugenyl acetate, up to 20% of b-caryophyllene, a-humulene, a-cubenene and a-copaene. [Perfumer & Flavourist (1978) Vol.2 No.7 pgs.44]

The recommended limit of use for pimento leaf oil and pimento berry oil is 4% and for clove leaf oil is 2%.

HIGH DERMAL TOXICITY
oregano oil (Origanum vulgare) Labiatae
[oral toxicity at 1.85g/kg & dermal toxicity at 0.48g/kg]
The United States NIOSH concurs with the RIFM on the oral toxicity value of oregano oil.
Several species of oregano are used for producing essential oils. The main species is the European oregano (O. vulgare). Other species include Italian oregano (O. gracile), Greek oregano (O. heracleoticum), Turkish oregano (O. smyrneaum), Syrian oregano (O. maru) and Moroccan oregano (O. virens). The plant called Spanish oregano (Thymus capitatus) is actually a species of thyme, similar to the other plant called Spanish marjoram (Thymus mastichiana).

Composition: 13.5% sabinene, 1.8% myrcene, 6.6% trans-2-hexenal, 13.5% cis-ocimene, 1.9% g-terpinene, 3.8% trans-ocimene, 3% p-cymene, 1.5% 3-octanol, 5.3% 1-octen-3-ol, 1.8% a-copaene, 3% linalool, 4.3% b-bourbonene, 9.2% caryophyllene, 1.2% aromadendrene, 1.4% a-humulene, 9.5% germacrene D, 3.4% bicyclogermacrene, 2.4% a-farnescene, 1.5% d-cadinene, 14% carvacrol and 12% thymol. [Perfumer & Flavourist (1989) Vol.14 No.1 pgs.36-9]

Italian oregano oil is very rich in thymol at 60% and Turkish oregano oil is very rich in carvacrol at 83% while Syrian oregano oil contains 44% carvacrol and 30% thymol. Greek oregano oil differs from the others in containing 13% p-cymene, 27% terpinen-4-ol, and only 18% thymol and 3% cavacrol. The oregano oils are not very important in flavouring and fragrance, used only in small quantities. [Perfumer & Flavourist (1977) Vol.2 No.7 pgs.48-9]

Commercial oregano oil is often mixed with that of Thymus capitatus; the sample tested by the RIFM was probably this commercial mixture.

savory oil, winter (Satureja hortensis) Labiatae
[oral toxicity at 1.37g/kg & dermal toxicity at 0.34g/kg]
The two main species of savory used for producing essential oils are the winter or garden savory (Satureja hortensis) and the summer or mountain savory (Satureja montana). Winter savory oil is mainly produced in France while Summer savory oil is produced in Spain. The chemical composition and odour of the two savory oils are very similar, summer savory oil being harsher than winter savory oil. The oils are valued for their fresh, herbaceous, spicy and slightly sharp phenolic notes due to their high content of carvacrol. Plant variations producing several chemotypes of oils occur but the classical composition of savory oil contains more carvacrol than thymol. [Perfumer & Flavourist (1978) Vol.3 No.6 pgs.57-8]

Composition: 60-75% carvacrol, 1-5% thymol, 10-20% p-cymene, 2-10% g-terpinene, 3.8% 1,8-cneole, 3% 1-octen-3-ol, 3.5% terpinen-4-ol, 12.5% borneol, 2.5% a-terpineol, 1.6% citronellal & carvone and 1% geraniol. [Perfumer & Flavourist (1981) Vol.6 No.4 pgs.76-77]

Applied at 100%, savory oil was strongly irritating to rabbit and guineapig skins and caused excoriation to mouse skin within 48 hours after application resulting in the death of half the number of test animals. At 10% it produced oedema. It was not irritating at 1% and below.

Recommended limit of use for oregano oil and savory oil is 0.5%.

Group I Grade 14 - carcinogenic potential

This category of essential oils contains principal constituents that are capable of inducing tumours when force-fed in large quantities over an extended period of time to test animals. Although the natural essential oils were not shown to be carcinogenic to humans, they are excluded from the approved lists of both the U.S. Food and Drug Administration and the Council of Europe. They are also not considered as GRAS by the Food Extracts Manufacturer's Association. Their value in aromatherapy is minimal and considering their potential hazards, are unsuitable for aromatherapy. **This category of essential oils is best not used.**

HEPATIC CARCINOGENS - Safrole containing essential oils (banned by the FDA in 1960)
The IFRA recommendation for essential oils containing safrole is not to use them at levels where the total safrole concentration exceeds 0.05%. The recommendation applies to sassafras oil, Brazilian sassafras oil, yellow camphor oil and brown camphor oil, all of which contain significant amounts of safrole. [IFRA Report Oct 76/Jul 87]

camphor oil, yellow (Cinnamomum camphora) Lauraceae
[oral toxicity at 3.85g/kg]
camphor oil, brown (Cinnamomum camphora) Lauraceae
[oral toxicity at 2.53g/kg]
Steam distillation of the wood of the camphor tree produces equal amounts of a crude camphor oil and a crystalline, translucent, semi-solid, white mass that sublimes on cooling. The crystalline camphor is separated out by filtration or by centrifuge and the crude oil is vacuum fractionated to yield three fractions: white, yellow and brown camphor oils. The safrole content of yellow and brown camphor oils is up to 80%.
[Perfumer & Flavourist (1979) Vol.4 No.4 pgs.49]

Brazilian sassafras oil (Ocotea cymbarum)* Lauraceae
[oral toxicity at 1.58g/kg]
Brazilian sassafras oil is steam distilled from the wood chips and sawdust of the tree growing in South America. The centre of production is in the Santa Catarina state of Brazil.

Composition: 60-90% safrole (the content of the main constituent is very variable), 3% camphone, 2% methyl eugenol, 0.3-0.6% eugenol and 0.2% 1,8-cineole.
[Perfumer & Flavourist (1985) Vol.10 No.4 pgs.48-51]

* Apparently, the correct botanical source of this essential oil is Ocotea pretiosa and not Ocotea cymbarum as was formerly thought.[de Matos Araujo 1945 & Mors, Taviera Magalhaes & Gottlieb 1959]
The RIFM used the name O. cymbarum and it is tentatively retained to avoid confusion.

Sassafras oil (Sassafras albidum) Lauraceae [oral toxicity at 1.9g/kg]

The sassafras tree is indigenous to North America growing wild over most of the central and eastern parts of the United States, very prolific in the Appalachian Mountain region. A tea brewed from sassafras root bark has been used for over 300 years in American folk medicine. Expeditions were made to North America to obtain sassafras for European use as early as 1574.

Various parts of the sassafras tree emit a characteristic spicy odour when crushed, the root-bark possessing the highest proportion of essential oil at 6 - 9%. Sassafras oil is produced by steam distillation of the root-bark mainly in the Appalachian region of Kentucky, Tennessee, North Carolina and Virginia with a smaller amount produced in southern Ohio and Indiana. It has always been a small volume item totalling about 20,000 lbs annually.

Sassafras oil had diverse uses in flavouring pharmaceutical preparations and semi-pharmaceuticals such as toothpastes and mouthwashes. It is also used to a limited extent in dentistry as a disinfectant in root canal work. Probably the best known use of sassafras oil is in flavouring sarsaparilla root-beer. [Perfumer & Flavourist (1979) Vol.3 No.6 pgs.31-2]

Composition: 60-80% safrole, 30% 5-methoxy-eugenol, 18% asarone, 11% piperonylacrolein, 7% coniferaldehyde, 5% camphone, and traces of menthone, thujone, anethole, apiole, elemicin, myristicin and eugenol. The hepatocarcinogenic metabolite, 1-hydroxy-safrole was not detected in sassafras oil. [Perfumer & Flavourist (1978) Vol.3 No.3 pgs.48]

Sassafras oil did not produce cross-sensitisation reactions in patients previously sensitised to Peru balsam, turpentine or colophony. It is reported to be carcinogenic in rats producing malignancy of the connective tissues, blood and lymphatic cells.

The Food Standards Committee recommendation for sassafras oil is that it should be prohibited for use in foods as a flavouring agent.[Report on flavouring agents (1965) HM Stationery Office, London]

Sassafras oil should not be taken internally. Large doses of sassafras oil cause fatty changes in the liver and kidneys. The use of sassafras tea may lead to a large dose of safrole.
[Martindale's Extra-Pharmacopoeia 28th ed. 1982]

The lethal oral dose of sassafras oil for a male adult is 1 teaspoonful. Cases of poisoning in children have been reported, the lethal oral dose for an infant is calculated as a few drops.

Although eugenol and anethole were known to be weak hepatotoxins, it appeared that safrole was the primary hepatocarcinogen. [Sethi, Subba, Chowdhury, Kapadia & Morton 1976]

However sassafras oil was reported to promote liver regeneration. [Gershbein 1977]

DUODENAL CARCINOGEN - Asarone containing essential oils(banned by the FDA in 1968) Presently calamus oil is the only one included in this category.

calamus oil (Acorus calamus) Araceae [oral toxicity at 0.77g/kg]

The United States NIOSH concurs with the RIFM on the oral toxicity value of calamus oil.

Calamus is a perennial, semi-aquatic, marshy plant native to northern Eurasia, ranging from Scotland across Europe, Russia, northern India and China to northern Japan. Calamus oil is obtained by steam distillation of either the fresh root or the unpeeled dried root, having a warm, spicy odour, reminiscent of a sweet forest. It has been widely used in flavours for liqueurs and vermouth as well as in perfumes.

Several chemical races of the calamus plant occur. Indian calamus is a tetraploid cultivar and the essential oil contains 82% b-asarone and 10% a-asarone; while European calamus is a diploid cultivar and the essential oil contains only 5% a-asarone and 0.2% b-asarone.

Composition of **European calamus oil**: 8% acorenone, 6.7% b-gurjunene, 6.2% isoshyobunone, 5.2% b-asarone, 5.2% calamendiol, 3.8% a-selinene, 3.5% a-calacorene, 3.2% calamusenone, 3.2% camphone, 2.6% shyobunone, 1.9% d-selinene, 1.7% d-cadinene, 1.5% camphene, 1.4% p-cymene, 1.4% carvacrol, 1.2% epishyobunone and 1% isocalamendiol.

Composition of **Indian calamus oil**: 77.7% b-asarone, 6.8% a-asarone, 1.3% cis-isoelemicin, 1.3% cis-methyl isoeugenol, 1% 2-furfural, 0.9% a-calacorene and 0.9% isocalamendiol.
[Perfumer & Flavourist (1986) Vol.11 No.3 pgs.52-4]

Calamus oil has been reported to cause dermatitis in hypersensitive individuals and to cause skin erythema when used in bath preparations. However it did not produce any sensitisation reactions when tested on 200 consecutive dermatitis patients or any cross-sensitisation when tested on 50 patients sensitive to Peru balsam, wood tars, colophony and turpentine.

Oral toxicity signs in rats include convulsions and severe liver and kidney damage, but test animals surviving for 3 days recovered completely from any liver or kidney damage. Daily oral doses at 0.25 - 2.0g/kg of food intake for 18 weeks caused liver and heart changes, the latter with slight myocardial degeneration characterised by muscle fibrosis and necrosis.

The calamus oil of commerce is from the Indian plant. In 1968, the b-asarone in Indian calamus oil was found to produce cancer in rats, however, in 1979, Japanese calamus oil which is obtained from a triploid cultivar containing 25% b-asarone and 8% a-asarone, was found not to be teratogenic to chickens after being injected into the eggs.
[Perfumer & Flavourist (1981) Vol.5 No.7 pgs.49-54]

Fed to rats at 0.05 - 0.5% in the daily diet, calamus oil caused malignant tumours to develop in the duodenum after 59 weeks.

Group I Grade 15 - very high oral and dermal toxicity

This category of essential oils is the most hazardous of all those tested by the RIFM in this series. The toxicity of bitter almond oil is due its content of benzaldehyde and particularly to the hydrocyanic acid. Removal of the hydrocyanic acid reduces the toxicity of the oil but it is still too hazardous for normal use. Chenopodium oil and boldo oil are the two most toxic of all the essential oils tested. They are both orally and dermally toxic at under 1g/kg corresponding to a theoretical toxic dose of <35 ml for a 70 kg adult. Both essential oils contain a high level of ascaridole which is responsible for their toxicity. Boldo oil having a greater oral-dermal toxicity differential than chenopodium oil is more topically hazardous while the latter is more systemically hazardous. The benefits of these essential oils are minimal while their hazards are great, they are therefore not suitable for aromatherapy and should be avoided.

almond oil, bitter (Prunus amygadalus) Rosaceae
[oral toxicity at 0.96g/kg & dermal toxicity at 1.2g/kg]
almond oil, bitter (Prunus amygadalus) Rosaceae [FFPA]
[oral toxicity at 1.5g/kg & dermal toxicity at >3g/kg]
The bitter almond tree is widely cultivated in Spain and North African countries including Morocco, Algeria, Tunisia and Egypt and also Turkey. The almond kernels are first separated from their shells and then crushed in a press. The spent shells are used in bakery ovens. The crushed kernels yield about 30% of fixed oil similar to sweet almond oil. The powdered cake left after pressing is then macerated in water to split the naturally occurring glycoside, amygdalin (mandelo-nitrile gentiobioside) by enzymatic action, and then distilled to yield 1% of the essential oil of bitter almond containing about 95% benzaldehyde and traces of hydrocyanic acid (formerly called prussic acid).

Human ingestion of 7.5 ml have been reported to result in death. Some bitter almond oil is treated with calcium hydroxide and ferrous sulphate to remove the hydrocyanic acid by separating out the blue precipitate, ferric ferrous cyanide. The oil is then redistilled filtered, dried and stored under nitrogen. This bitter almond oil is termed FFPA - free from prussic acid.

Bitter almond oil rapidly oxidises to benzoic acid forming white crystals around the caps of containers. It is highly recommended that 10% of ethanol which has a stabilising effect on the benzaldehyde be added to bitter almond oil and then store under nitrogen. When well-stored, it should keep for a year. The natural oil was given GRAS status by the FEMA in 1965 and is approved for food use by the FDA and the Council of Europe in 1974. It is used extensively to flavour marzipans, persipans and macaroons. [Perfumer & Flavourist (1991) Vol.16 No.6 pgs.17-24]

Almond oil has been known to cause dermatitis in sensitive individuals.

chenopodium oil (Chenopodium ambrosioides) Chenopodiaceae
[oral toxicity at 0.25g/kg & dermal toxicity at 0.414g/kg]

Chenopodium also known as wormseed is a plant native to North America. The whole plant is steam distilled to produce an essential oil. Chenopodium has been a small crop in the United States for over 100 years, cultivated primarily in Maryland with some production in the central Ohio valley. Production of the essential oil has declined recently from approximately 100,000 lbs from 18 distillers in 1935 to just 4000 lbs from 2 distillers in 1978.
[Perfumer & Flavourist (1979) Vol.3 No.6 pgs.28]

Chenopodium oil is pale yellow in colour with a characteristic unpleasant odour and a bitter burning taste. The natural oil contains not less than 65% ascaridole. It has been used for the expulsion of roundworms (ascarids) and hookworms. However, it is toxic to the liver and kidneys being replaced by less toxic drugs and is contra-indicated in patients with impaired liver or kidney function and the debilitated. In the early part of the 20th century, chenopodium oil was quite important as it was one of the best known natural anthelmintics being successfully used throughout Europe and the British Commonwealth.

Several cases of fatal human poisoning by chenopodium oil have been reported. Cumulative effects may be produced by small doses given several days apart. Toxic effects include skin and mucous membrane irritation, headache, vertigo, nausea, vomiting, constipation, tinnitus, temporary deafness, diplopia (double vision) and blindness, transient stimulation followed by depression of the central nervous system leading to delirium and coma, occasional convulsions, circulatory collapse due to vasomotor paralysis and sometimes pulmonary oedema.

Toxic epidermal necrolysis has been reported after the ingestion of chenopodium oil.
[Archs Derm (1960) 82/903]

The ascaridole in chenopodium oil is an unstable compound and may cause it to explode when heated or treated with organic acids. [Martindale's Extra-Pharmacopoeia 28th ed. 1982]

boldo oil (Peumus boldus) Monimiaceae
[oral toxicity at 0.13g/kg & dermal toxicity at 0.9g/kg]

The essential oil of boldo is steam distilled from the leaves of the boldo tree growing wild in South America, particularly in Chile. Boldo oil is not a very popular fragrance ingredient but a few perfumers seem to like its unique fragrance characteristics.

Composition: 28.6% p-cymene, 4% a-pinene, 0.8% b-pinene, 1.6% limonene, 1% g-terpinene, 0.8% sabinene, 0.6% camphene, 0.5% d-3-carene, 0.4% terpinolene, 16% ascaridole, 9% linalool, 2.6% terpinen-4-ol, 0.9% a-terpineol, 0.9% fenchol, 0.8% fenchone, 0.6% camphone, 0.4% farnesol, 0.4% 2-nonanone, 0.5% methyl eugenol, 0.3% cuminaldehyde and 0.5% coumarin. [Perfumer & Flavourist (1977) vol.2 No.1 pgs.3]

An oral dose of 0.07g/kg in rats produced convulsions with death occurring at 0.13g/kg.

Group II - concretes and absolutes

Concretes and absolutes are not normally used in aromatherapy due to the presence of trace amounts of solvents left in them during the extraction process. They generally tend to cause more adverse reactions on the skin than their corresponding distilled essential oils. However only concretes and absolutes can be obtained from plants whose floral parts would not yield to distillation. There the corresponding essential oils will not be available. If their therapeutic properties are desired in therapy, the absolutes may be used. Concretes are less pure than absolutes and are also solid. They are generally not suitable for use in aromatherapy.

USEFUL FLORAL ABSOLUTES - Grade 1 & 2

neroli/orange flower absolute (Citrus aurantium) Rutaceae - 20%
jasmine absolute (Jasminum officinale) Oleaceae - 3%
rose absolute, French (Rosa centifolia) Rosaceae - 2%

The RIFM determined the dermal toxicity value of rose absolute from an 'inadequate sample' as >0.8g/kg. Test results for the rose oils were more reliable and rose absolute is tentatively assumed to have a comparable dermal toxicity value with rose oil.

These three floral absolutes are the most commonly used in aromatherapy. Two of these floral absolutes, neroli and jasmine have Grade 1 dermal toxicity at 5g/kg while rose absolute has Grade 2 dermal toxicity at 2.5g/kg.

Jasmine flowers are traditionally not distilled and only the absolute is available. Among the absolutes, it is comparatively mild and non-toxic and has been used by some aromatherapists for treatments without any adverse effects. Rose and neroli absolutes are generally not used in aromatherapy since their distilled essential oils are available and preferable for use in treatments. The only advantge of the absolutes is their lower cost compared to the price of floral essential oils. All three absolutes are safe at a concentration of 2 - 3%, neroli absolute has also been shown to be safe at up to 20%.

Modern advanced extraction techniques can now provide jasmine essential oil extracted by liquid carbon dioxide without using any organic solvents and avoiding the problem of trace contaminants in the final product. When obtainable, it is preferable to the absolute for use in treatments.

USEFUL LEAF ABSOLUTE - Grade 1
Violet leaf absolute is presently the only one in this category.

violet leaf absolute (Viola odorata) Violaceae - 2% *[not tested for toxicity]*

The RIFM did not test violet leaf absolute for oral or dermal toxicity and presently this information is not available elsewhere. However it has been used in aromatherapy at the usual 2% without any adverse effects and appears to be similarly mild like jasmine absolute.

Composition of **violet flower absolute**: 2-trans-6-cis-nonadien-1-al, n-hexanol, heptenol, octadienal, benzyl alcohol, eugenol, decanone-2, isoborneol, zingiberene, b-curcumene, dihydro-a-ionone, dihydro-b-ionone, a-ionone, b-ionone, vanillin and diethyl phthalate.
Composition of **violet leaf absolute**: 2-trans-6-cis-nonadien-1-al, n-hexanol, n-octen-2-ol-1, benzyl alcohol, tertiary octenol, hexenol, heptenol, octenol and traces of eugenol.
No quantitative data was available. [Perfumer & Flavourist (1978) Vol.3 No.1 pgs29-32]

The odour of violet is mainly due to the compound, 2-trans-6-cis-nonadien-1-al, which occurs in a higher concentration in the leaves than in the flowers. While nonadienal and nonedienol are largely responsible for the odour of violet flowers and leaves, small amounts of ionones and dihydro-ionones contribute to the floral note of the violet scent. Violet notes contribute an important role in the formulation of fine fragrances.

The following absolutes are comparable to the Grade 1 essential oils with minimal hazard potential. However, they have only minor importance in aromatherapy, their corresponding essential oils being available and preferable.

lavandin absolute (Lavandula hybrida) Labiatae - 10%
lavender absolute (Lavandula officinalis) Labiatae - 10%
[oral toxicity at 4.52g/kg] *[not tested for phototoxicity]*
Lavender absolute has been listed as a sensitiser.

olibanum absolute (Boswellia carterii) Burseraceae - 8%
[not tested for toxicity] The RIFM did not test olibanum absolute for oral or dermal toxicity. They are tentatively assumed to be comparable to that of olibanum gum.

eau de brouts absolute (Citrus aurantium) Rutaceae - 4%
Eau de brouts is extracted from a mixture of petitgrain and neroli.

labdanum absolute (Cistus ladaniferus) Cistaceae - 4%
A greenish alcoholic extract with a sweet, amber-like odour.

immortelle absolute (Helichrysum angustifolium) Compositae - 2%
[oral toxicity at 4.4g/kg]

foin absolute (Anthoxanthum odoratum) Graminae - 4%

The following absolutes are also comparable to the Grade 1 essential oils except fenugreek absolute which has grade 2 dermal toxicity. This category of absolutes does not have the corresponding essential oils commercially available. However they are of minimal importance and are not normally used in aromatherapy.

orris root absolute (Iris pallida) Iridaceae - 3% *[not tested for dermal toxicity]*

The oral toxicity of orris root absolute was determined by the RIFM to be comparatively low at 9.4g/kg. When retested at 100% for 24 hours, orris root absolute did not produce any irritation reactions. The absolute of orris root resembles the absolutes of violet in odour and also contains ionones. Orris root absolute is not as important as violet leaf absolute in aromatherapy. It is also much more expensive.

Powdered orris is yellowish-white to pale yellow in colour. It may cause allergic reactions in hypersensitive individuals. [Martindale's Extra-Pharmacopoeia 28th ed. 1982]

deertongue absolute (Liatris odoratissima) Compositae - 5%

Deertongue is a plant native to the southeastern United States. The plant does not contain any appreciable essential oil, however, a rich, sweet, powdery, herbaceous, coumarin-like extract can be obtained from the leaves. The absolute is not used in flavouring due to its coumarin content and has only a limited use in fragrances.

genet absolute (Spartium junceum) Leguminosae - 12%

Genet is also called broom in English as the plant's twigs were used as brooms for sweeping. The plant grows wild in the Mediterranean countries. The yellow-golden flowers possess a dusty-sweet odour reminiscent of orange blossoms and grape. Genet flower absolute is viscous and dark brown in colour. It is produced in the Grasse region of southern France and in Italy. A steam distilled concrete yielding the essential oil is only used for scientific research. Genet absolute is warm, harsh and very long lasting but is considered slightly too green and therefore requires the addition of sweeteners. It is classified in the tuberose-narcissus group. Benzoin and storax resinoids, labdanum and vetivert oils, orris and oakmoss concretes and Tolu balsam are used as fixatives for the genet scent. Both genet absolute and concrete of French and Italian origin are still commercially available and they remain valuable perfumery materials. Genet absolute imparts a special cachet to heavier fragrances. It blends especially well with orange flower absolute and is also useful in linden blossom blends up to 1%.
[Perfumer & Flavourist (1991) Vol.16 No.5 pgs.55-7]

Composition: 2% ethyl myristate, 14.56% ethyl palmitate, 3.6% ethyl stearate, 4.8% ethyl oleate, 7% ethyl linoleate, 1.5% methyl linolenate, 3.4% linalyl acetate, 3.2% 1-octen-3-ol, 11% linalool, 1.3% phenyl ethyl alcohol, 1.7% b-farnescene, 4% capric acid, 2.9% myristic acid, 20.9% palmitic acid, 3.5% stearic acid, 5.85% oleic acid, 4.6% linoleic acid and 15.7% linolenic acid. [Perfumer & Flavourist (1981) Vol.6 No.2 pgs.60]

fenugreek absolute (Trigonella foenum-graecum) Leguminosae - 2%

Numerous types of fenugreek extracts are available. The extracts are generally prepared by initially extracting the ground seeds with alcohol. Most of the differences between the extracts relate to the timing of the heat treatments of the seeds up to roasting temperatures prior to extraction. Extracts of fenugreek have been used as flavouring ingredients. They are used in fragrance composition only to a small extent.

Composition: 5-10% hexanol & heptanoic acid, 0.5-5% heptanal, with 1,8-cineole, dodecene, decanoic acid, dihydro-benzofuran, hexyl furan, g-nonalactone, tetradecene, a-muurolene, z-muurolene, g-muurolene, b-elemene and calamenene.
[Perfumer & Flavourist (1987) Vol.12 No.5 pgs.60]

tobacco leaf absolute (Nicotiana affinis) Solanaceae - 1%

Cured tobacco leaves are extracted with petroleum ether to produce the concrete which is then extracted with alcohol to yield the dark-brown semi-solid absolute. Tobacco concrete and absolute are relatively new perfumery materials. The extracts are solvent extracted under sophisticated conditions from dried tobacco leaf dust, crumbs and stalks to produce a yield between 0.2-2%. The tobacco scent is used in the fragrance industry to depict harmony as well as a pleasant note in masculine fragrances. [Perfumer & Flavourist (1984) Vol.9 No.5 pgs.62]

MILD PHOTOTOXIC POTENTIAL

honeysuckle absolute (Lonicera caprifolium) Caprifoliaceae - 3%

[not tested for toxicity] The RIFM did not test honeysuckle absolute for oral or dermal toxicity. This information is presently not available elsewhere. **Uncertain toxicity.**
Honeysuckle absolute possesses minimal phototoxic potential tested at 100% but is not phototoxic below 50% diluted in benzene or below 70% in methanol.

The honeysuckle plant originated in Asia Minor, but is now cultivated in many countries of the world. Steam distillation of the flowers produces an essential oil with a yellowish colour. The composition of the oil is presently not well known but appears not to contain any aldehydes, ketones or nitrogenous compounds. A viscous, olive-green absolute is produced in the south of France in small quantities for using in deluxe fragrances. Like lily-of-the-valley and lilac, it is very difficult to obtain sufficient quantities of honeysuckle extracts. The honeysuckle scent can be considered in both the narcissus or the jasmine groups. In basic compounding, the honeysuckle fragrance is built on lily-of-the-valley components combined with constituents of jasmine and rose, especially their alcohols. Additionally, components of neroli and ylang-ylang are also included, as well as jasmine, rose, tuberose, mimosa and violet leaf absolutes in small amounts. The fixatives used for honeysuckle compounds include Tolu balsam, storax and olibanum. Honeysuckle is very seldom used as a fragrance on its own. It serves mostly as a valuable component in blends. Fine fragrances with honeysuckle as an ingredient include Quelques Fleurs, Couer de Jeanette, Tatiana, Sikkim, Christian Aujart, Premiere and Crystalle.
[Perfumer & Flavourist (1989) Vol.14 No.5 pgs.19-22]

MODERATE DERMAL TOXICITY

hyacinth absolute (Hyacinthus orientalis) Liliaceae - 8%
Hyacinth originated in Asia Minor and spread into cultivation in Europe in the 15th century. It was cultivated in southern France and in Holland in the early 1920's. Some hyacinth also grows wild in the south of France. The wild flowers have a more floral and fresher scent than the flowers of cultivated hyacinth. Both French and Dutch hyacinth flowers are used for extracting absolutes, the Dutch type having a greener and more powerful odour than the French. In recent times, hyacinth absolute production has almost ceased in both France and Holland and synthetic compounds have been developed for the hyacinth scent using fixatives including galbanum resin, storax resinoid, Tolu balsam and guaiacwood oil. A combination of rose, jasmine, lilac and lily-of-the-valley components can be used to reproduce the hyacinth scent. Hyacinth absolute when available is used in high class fragrances and other floral perfumes including Nuance by Coty, Votre by Jourdan, Grain de Sable by Verfaillie, Cabriole by Arden, Tanago by Leonard, Pavlova by Payot, Cristalle by Chanel, Azzaro and Armani.
[Perfumer & Flavourist (1986) Vol.10 No.6 pgs.17-20]

Composition: 8% benzyl acetate, 40% benzyl alcohol, 1.5% methyl eugenol, 3% trimethoxybenzene, 11% trans-cinnamyl alcohol, 1.2% phenyl ethyl alcohol and 1.2% phenyl ethyl benzoate. [Perfumer & Flavourist (1978) Vol.3 No.2 pgs.46]

The juice of hyacinth bulbs has powerful skin irritating properties, with reported cases of generalised eczema covering almost the entire skin, with dry, scaly and fissured lesions at the finger tips and itching behind both ears. Dermatoses produced by handling the bulbs have been reported among sorters and packers in nursery gardens.

MODERATE ORAL AND DERMAL TOXICITY

karo karounde absolute (Leptactina senegambica) Rubiaceae - 1%
[oral toxicity at 1.4g/kg]
Karo karounde absolute is first solvent extracted from the flowers of a plant native to tropical Africa, with hexane to yield the concrete and further treated with alcohol to obtain the viscous, dark orange-brown absolute with an intensely floral, herbaceous, sweet odour. The major bulk of the absolute consists of saturated and unsaturated fatty acids, together with their ethyl, 2-methylbutyl, benzyl and phenylethyl esters.

tonka absolute (Dipteryx odorata) Leguminosae - 8%
The tonka tree is native to tropical America and tonka absolute is extracted from the seeds. It is a semi-solid or crystalline mass of pale amber (brownish-yellow) colour with a coumarinic, herbaceous odour. Its main constituent is coumarin. The fragrant seeds are also cured in rum and used for scenting tobacco and snuff.

deertongue incolore (Liatris odoratissima) Compositae - 5%
[oral toxicity at 0.73g/kg & dermal toxicity at 3.67g/kg]
The incolore is the absolute decolourised by charcoal. When deertongue absolute is decolourised, the toxicity, both oral and dermal is increased significantly.

Minimal therapeutic importance. Maintain low concentrations not exceeding 1%

IRRITATION AND SENSITISATION POTENTIAL

mastic absolute (Pisticia lentiscus) Anacardiaceae - 8%
Mastic pollen extracts did not produce any irritation reactions when tested in non-atopic patients but when tested on 58 atopic patients, they produced 16 irritation reactions. Mastic absolute has been reported to be a sensitiser.

verbena absolute (Lippia citriodora) Verbenaceae - 2%
Verbena absolute did not produce any irritation reactions when tested at 12% on 26 volunteers but produced 3 sensitisation reactions. When it was tested at 2%, it did not produce any sensitisation reactions.

narcissus absolute (Narcissus poetieus) Amaryllidaceae - 2%
jonquil absolute (Narcissus jonquilla) Amaryllidaceae - 2%
[not tested for toxicity] Jonquil absolute was not tested by the RIFM for oral or dermal toxicity. They are tentatively assumed to be similar to that of narcissus absolute.
The narcissus plant has been reported to be a sensitiser.

Composition of narcissus: 14% benzyl alcohol, 13.7% benzyl acetate, 16% linalool, 12.5% indole, 8.3% heneicosane, 5.5% a-terpineol, 4.4% methoxy phenyl ethyl acetate, 1.8% phenyl propyl acetate, 1.5% phenyl ethyl acetate, 1% methoxy benzyl acetate, 1% 1,8-cineole and 1% limonene. [Perfumer & Flavourist (1992) Vol.17 No.4 pgs.39-42]

The absolutes of narcissus and jonquil are obtained from the flowers. They are both important in perfumery for their rich fragrances resembling a combination of rose, orange flowers, jasmine, ylang-ylang, tuberose, violets and orris. Narcissus absolute is used as a component of Silences by Jacomo and jonquil absolute is used as a component of Nuance by Coty. Both absolutes are used in traces in Je Reviens by Worth.

mimosa absolute (Acacia decurrens) Leguminosae - 1%
Mimosa absolute may produce dermatitis in hypersensitive individuals.

Minimal therapeutic importance. Moderate risk of irritation and sensitisation, maintain low concentrations not exceeding 1%. Avoid using on hypersensitive individuals.

CROSS-SENSITISATION POTENTIAL

The three fragrance materials in this category possess cross-sensitisation potential. Their toxicity varies slightly among themselves. Benzoin resinoid has Grade 1 toxicity and vanilla tincture has Grade 2 toxicity. The oral and dermal toxicity of myrrh absolute however were not determined by the RIFM. They are tentatively assumed to be similar to that of myrrh oil which has a dermal toxicity of 5g/kg and an oral toxicity value of 1.65g/kg (Grade 6 toxicity).

vanilla tincture (Vanilla planifolia) Orchidaceae - 10%

Unlike an absolute, the alcohol in not removed from the tincture and the final product is kept in an alcoholic solution similar to the herbal preparation. The essential oil of vanilla is always prepared as a tincture, even when sometimes sold as an 'essence'. According to the U.S. Food and Drug Administration, vanilla tincture is a solution containing no less than 35% alcohol. The main country of vanilla production is Mexico. Vanilla tincture did not produce any irritation reactions when tested at 100% on 31 volunteers. When tested on 73 patients sensitive to Peru balsam, vanilla tincture produced 34 cross-sensitisation reactions, however, patients sensitive to vanilla tincture did not react positively when tested with Peru balsam.

Composition: caproic acid, guaiacol, b-phenyl ethyl alcohol, heptanoic acid, creosol, octanoic acid, g-nonalactone, p-cresol, trans-methyl cinnamate, nonanoic acid, eugenol, vanillyl ethyl ether, anisaldehyde, furfural, methyl palmitate, ethyl palmitate, anisyl ethyl ether, anisyl acetate, anisyl alcohol, methyl anisate, cis-methyl cinnamate and vanillin. **No quantitative data was available.** [Perfumer & Flavourist (1977) Vol.2 No.1 pgs.6-7]

benzoin resinoid (Styrax benzoin) Styracaceae - 8%

[not tested for phototoxicity] Benzoin resinoid is obtained by extracting the natural benzoin with benzene and then distilling off the solvent. The resinoid is not treated again with alcohol. Sometimes benzoin is also prepared as a mixed tincture together with other fragrance materials. Benzoin resinoid did not produce any irritation reactions when tested at 8% and is not itself a sensitiser. In the concentrations and forms employed in toilet preparations, benzoin is not a primary irritant. However, tincture of benzoin that also contains storax resinoid and Peru and Tolu balsams, produced cross-sensitisation to the two balsams.

myrrh absolute (Commiphora myrrha) Burseraceae - 8%

[not tested for toxicity] Myrrh absolute was not tested by the RIFM for oral or dermal toxicity.
Tested in a patient who developed contact dermatitis to benzoin tincture followed by non-eczematous eruption, myrrh absolute produced cross-sensitisation reactions.

Vanilla tincture is not suitable for aromatherapy use due to its high alcohol content, and myrrh absolute is not important as myrrh essential oil is available and is preferable. Benzoin resinoid is not available as a pure essential oil so is used as a resinoid in aromatherapy. Avoid using this group of fragrance materials with others that they can cross-sensitise especially the Group 3 materials: gums, resins and balsams. Limit to 3%.

STRONG SENSITISATION POTENTIAL

costus root absolute & concrete (Saussurea lappa) Compositae

Extracts of costus root, both the absolute and concrete, are strong sensitisers even at 2%, producing very severe positive sensitisation reactions in some test volunteers.

The recommendation for costus root absolute and concrete is that it should not be used.
The IFRA recommendation for costus root absolute and concrete is similar to their recommendation for costus root oil based on the RIFM test results showing sensitising potential in some samples and absence of sensitising potential in other samples.

STRONG PHOTOTOXIC POTENTIAL

fig leaf absolute (Ficus carica) Moraceae

Fig leaf absolute is a relatively rare fragrance raw material. It is obtained by hydrocarbon extraction followed by alcohol wash of the fig leaves. The absolute is dark green, viscous liquid or semi-solid with a delicately sweet, green, herbaceous, woody fragrance with mossy undertones.

The composition of fig leaf absolute consisting of 3 fractions was determined in 1986:
73% residue fraction composed of a mixture of resinous materials
26% non-volatile fraction composed of fatty acids and their ethyl esters
 1% nitrogenous fraction composed of 29% 2-siobutyl-4-methylpyridine, 10% 2-isobutanoyl-4-methylpyridine, 6% 2-isobytenyl-4-methylpyridine, 4% 2-methyl-propyl-4-methylpyridine, 4% quinoline, 2.2% dimethyl-leucine methyl ester, 1.5% dimethyl-anthranilate and 1.5% cinamonitrile. [Perfumr & Flavourist (1988) Vol.13 No.6 pgs.58-60]
(The main component of a vacuum distilled fig leaf extract is 56% germacrene D)

Fig leaves contain furocoumarins which cause phototoxicity and fresh fig fruits have also been reported to be photosensitising. Fig leaf absolute has been reported as a sensitiser and to cause phototoxic reactions on human skin. [Kaiser 1986]

It has strong phototoxicity from 12.5% and even at a concentration as low as 0.001% it still produces phototoxic reactions in half the number of test animals. Tested at 5% on 25 volunteers, fig leaf absolute produced 1 irritation reaction and 2 sensitisation reactions.

The IFRA recommendation for fig leaf absolute is that it should not be used as a fragrance ingredient. This recommendation is based on the RIFM test results showing sensitisation and extreme phototoxic potential for this fragrance material.
[IFRA Revised Amendments Annex 1 June 1979]

SENSITISATION AND CROSS-SENSITISATION POTENTIAL

Concretes unlike absolutes and essential oils are solids. They are important in perfumery as fixatives but have minimal value in aromatherapy. These two concretes from mosses are not suitable for aromatherapy treatments because of their sensitisation and cross-sensitisation hazards.

treemoss concrete (Usnea barbata) Usneaceae [oral toxicity at 4.33g/kg]
oakmoss concrete (Evernia prunastri) Usneaceae [oral toxicity at 2.9g/kg]
The various extracts of mosses (concretes, absolutes & resinoids) are used in perfumery to lend naturalness and body, rich pleasant undertones and high fixative values in numerous types of fragrances. These mosses are lichens that grow on trees. The oakmoss grows primarily on oak trees and is collected all over central and southern Europe, particularly in France and Yugoslavia and also in north Africa in Algeria and Morocco. The treemoss grows on other trees especially spruces, firs and pines in the humid forests of central and southern Europe. In China, several species of treemosses have since 1960 been harvested from the Yunnan province for extracting the concretes. There, a related species of oakmoss, E. mesomorpha, grows on agalea trees at an altitude between 27 - 42000 metres and two other species of treemosses, Ramalina fastigiata and Cetrariastrum nepalensis are also found. Among the three moss absolutes, the Chinese oakmoss absolute has the finest and most pronounced odour resembling the European oakmoss absolute, while the R. fastigiata absolute is much less refined and the C. nepalensis absolute is more tender and greenish. All three absolutes are used in the Chinese perfumery industry for their fixative properties. [Perfumer & Flavourist (1988) Vol.13. No.5 pgs.13-6]

Tree mosses or lichens are among the voluminous botanicals which are solvent extracted for use in perfumery. Before extraction, the lichens with a natural moisture content of about 12% are humidified by spraying with hot water and kept wet overnight for fermentation to occur increasing the temperature to around 40 - 50 degrees C. in the centre of the bulk. The moisture restores the cell wall permeability and makes the solvent extraction easier. It also prevents spore dust from dispersing in the production area. Fermentation causes the hydrolysis of dipsides that are responsible for the odour of mosses. The extraction process traditionally takes over 12 hours. [Perfumer & Flavourist (1990) Vol.15 No.6 pgs.15-6]

The main problem with the moss concretes is that they vary considerably among suppliers. The origin of the raw material and the processing conditions are mainly responsible for this situation. It is also common practice to mix raw materials with moss extracts, and they are known in the trade to be the most compounded of all the natural fragrance extracts available. **The IFRA recommendation for treemoss and oakmoss extracts (concretes, absolutes and resinoids) obtained from Usnea and Evernia species is that they should not be used individually or in combination such that the level exceeds 0.6% in a consumer product and 3% in a fragrance compound**. This recommendation is based on the RIFM test results showing the sensitising and cross-reactivity potentials of oakmoss and treemoss extracts.
[IFRA Guidelines 1992]

Group III - gums, resins and balsams

The main hazards with gums, resins and balsams is cross-sensitisation reactions to any of them in individuals already sensitised to another such substance or to benzoin resinoid. Most fragrance materials are highly volatile and do not have prolonged retention times on the skin to penetrate the stratum corneum slowly in order to induce sensitisation reactions. However, some fragrance materials polymerise and provide enough residence time on the skin to become sensitisers. The most notable are found in the small group of gums, resins and balsams which contain the greatest amounts of polymers. The RIFM tests seemed to show a pattern among both adverse reaction accounts and reported sensitisers. Moreover, when this group of fragrance materials is distilled through high vacuum to remove their non-volatile residue, they yield their respective essential oils that are markedly less active as allergens than the crude gums, resins and balsams.
[Hjorth (1961) Aarhuus Stiftsbogtrykkerie]

olibanum gum (Boswellia carterii) Burseraceae - 8%
[not tested for phototoxicity] Olibanum is also known by the Biblical name of 'frankincense'

galbanum resin (Ferula galbaniflua) Umbelliferae - 8%
Galbanum resin did not produce any irritation reactions when tested at 2 - 20% on healthy volunteers and at 0.1% on dermatosis patients. Tested on a patient who developed contact dermatitis followed by non-eczematous eruptions to benzoin tincture, galbanum resin produced cross-sensitisation reactions.

fir balsam, Canadian (Abies balsamea) Pinaceae *[not tested for phototoxicity]*
Canadian fir balsam is a pale yellow viscous oleoresin with an agreeable odour and a bitter, acrid taste. It is often used in microscopy as a mounting medium.

Douglas fir balsam (Pseudotsuga taxifolia) Pinaceae - 8%
Douglas fir balsam is light amber-coloured and collected either from the trunks of felled trees or by inserting a tube into live trees.

gurjun balsam (Dipterocarpus turbinatus) Dipterocarpaceae - 8%
Gurjun balsam is the oleoresin exuded by incision from the tree trunks composed almost entirely of the essential oil at 60 - 80% and gurjunic acid resin.

copaiba balsam (Copaifera reticulata) Leguminosae - 8%
Copaiba balsam is collected by tapping the trees and contains substantial quantities of the essential oil with small quantities of resin and acids.

Peru balsam (Myroxylon pereirae) Leguminosae

Peru balsam is a dark brown viscous oleoresin exuded from the trunk of the tree with an agreeable balsamic odour and a bitter, burning taste. It contains 50 - 60% of balsamic esters.

Peru balsam may cause skin sensitisation. [Martindale's Extra-Pharmacopoeia 28th ed. 1982]
Of 4000 patients subjected to Peru balsam patch testing at 25% in five European clinics, 184 males and 304 females showed positive reactions. [H. Bandmann, Archs Derm (1972) 106/335]

Tested at 8% on 25 volunteers by the RIFM, Peru balsam produced 7 sensitisation reactions. It is reported to be among the most common allergens causing cross-sensitisation reactions in individuals sensitised to poplar resin.

The IFRA recommendation for Peru balsam is not to use as a fragrance ingredient but to use Peru balsam oil (extracted by distillation) instead which is free from allergens. This recommendation is based on the RIFM test results showing the sensitisation potential of Peru balsam and the absence of sensitisation potential of Peru balsam oil and compounds containing Peru balsam oil.

Tolu balsam (Myroxylon balsamum) Leguminosae - 2%

[not tested for phototoxicity]
Tolu balsam is a soft, tenacious, brownish-yellow oleoresin when fresh, obtained by incision of the trunk of the tree, subsequently becoming harder and finally brittle, with a vanilla like odour and taste. It contains 35 - 50% of balsamic acids.

Tolu balsam did not produce any irritation or sensitisation reactions when tested at 100% for 48 hours in a patient with perfume dermatitis. In tests conducted on 67 patients sensitised to Peru balsam, Tolu balsam tested in alcohol at 10% for 10 tests produced cross-sensitisation reactions in 50% of the patients and at 1% for 27 tests produced cross-sensitisation reactions in 73% of the patients. Tested as a powder in vaseline at 5% Tolu balsam only produced cross-sensitisation reactions in 21% of the patients. Positive reactions were more frequent with alcoholic solutions.

Sensitivity to Tolu balsam is always accompanied by sensitivity to Peru balsam and benzoin and the constituents coniferyl benzoate and coniferyl cinnamate. Among the crude fragrance materials tested, Peru balsam contains the highest residue content (30 - 40%) and is the most notorious sensitiser. The sensitising potential of Peru balsam is shared by Tolu balsam, galbanum and opoponax.

Gums, resins and balsams are crude aromatics and are not normally used in aromatherapy except perhaps for burning as dry incense. When used as such, they do not come into direct contact with the skin and the concentration of their vapours in the air is usually quite low. For using on the skin, the respective essential oils purified from this group of raw fragrance materials are less hazardous and preferable to the crude exudates.

Spurious essential oils

The essential oils in this category are unusual fragrant by-products of other materials. They have a limited use in perfumery but have no importance in the practice of aromatherapy.

cognac oil, green (Vitis vinifera) Vitidaceae
Cognac oil is not really a true essential oil. It is obtained from the steam distillation of wine sediments (grape residue and yeast) from which the alcoholic beverage has been distilled. Chemically, cognac oil consists of a number of ethyl esters and isomyl esters: ethyl hexanoate, ethyl heptanoate, ethyl octanoate, ethyl decanoate, ethyl laurate, ethyl myristate & ethyl palmitate. [Perfumer & Flavourist (1978) Vol.3 No.6 pgs.55]

ale oil (Pinus sp.) Pinaceae
Ale oil is extracted from pine wood during the sulphate paper process as a by-product of the wood-pulp industry.

This group of essential oils are not normally used in aromatherapy.

Modified fragrance materials

The chemical composition of these essential oils has been altered to produce a change of odour for perfumery preferences. In the acetylated form, they do not occur in nature and are no longer suitable for aromatherapy use where the natural constitution of the essential oil is paramount. Their corresponding natural essential oils are available and should be used instead.

amyris oil [acetylated]
bois de rose oil [acetylated]
(Eucalyptus citriodora) oil [acetylated]
lavandin absolute [acetylated]

Acetylation is the process of increasing the ester content of organic compounds, especially those containing alcohols, by introducing anhydride to form the acetates.

Simply avoid this type of fragrance materials in aromatherapy.

Chapter 8

Supplement on Fragrance Materials without RIFM monographs

There are still several other essential oils of interest to aromatherapy that do not yet have monographs of safety information published for them by the RIFM. These include peppermint oil, melissa oil, wild thyme oil, yarrow oil, santolina oil, valerian oil, olibanum oil, galangal oil and amyris oil. Until further information on their safety becomes available, tentative estimations have been made for their safety application based on a combination of their botanical affinity and their chemical nature together with any clinical or other related information. These estimations are assumed to be applicable for the meantime.

Many other essential oils and absolutes have already been studied and described. Some are becoming better known because of their published studies. These include spikenard oil, agarwood oil, tejpat oil, zdravetz oil and buchu oil. Others are still quite obscure, especially those from less accessible tropical regions of the world. However they have already gained the attention of the fragrance materials market and may become more important in the future. When there is no basis for estimating their safety application, no attempt has been made at speculation.

Several very rare floral essential oils that have featured historically in the development of perfumery but could not be produced in sufficient quantities to be of more widespread usefulness, are also included with background information for the awareness of readers. These include lily-of-the-valley oil, lilac oil, gardenia oil, mignonette oil, carnation oil, cassie oil, magnolia oil, osmanthus oil and tuberose absolute. No attempt has been made to evaluate their safety application. They remain of academic interest only.

A few essential oils are sufficiently well documented to allow their safety application to be determined without the benefit of any RIFM safety monographs. These include wintergreen oil, mustard oil, horseradish oil and savin oil.

In total, an additional 60 essential oils and absolutes that have been documented are included in this chapter together with available botanical, chemical and background information to supplement the 190 already described in Chapter 7.

peppermint oil (Mentha piperita) Labiatae

The United States NIOSH determined the oral toxicity of peppermint oil to be 4.44g/kg (rat) Peppermint oil may cause allergic reactions. [Martindale Extra-Pharmacopoeia 28th ed. 1982]

2 patients addicted to peppermint sucking suffered from idiopathic auricular fibrillation, normal rhythm was restored when the sucking ceased. [Lancet (1962) 1, 222]

Using a toothpaste containing peppermint oil was reported to cause an acute allergic reaction in the mouth, throat and neck. [Br dent J (1968) 125, 304]

2 patients consuming large quantities of confectionery flavoured with peppermint oil suffered from recurrent attacks of muscle pain. [Med J Aust (1972) 2, 390]

Safety applications for peppermint oil can be tentatively assumed to be comparable to that of spearmint oil with a **recommended limit of use at 4%** until further information becomes available from the RIFM. **Reduce to 0.1% for hypersensitive individuals.**

melissa oil (Melissa officinalis) Labiatae

Melissa is a species related to the mints found from Europe to Central Asia. The plant can be steam distilled to produce an essential oil. However the yield is extremely low and many oils offered commercially are adulterated with other essential oils, essential oil constituents or even synthetic chemicals. Consequently, the genuine oil is very much more expensive.

principal constituents	French (fresh)	French (dried)	German (fresh)	Indian (fresh)	Canadian (fresh)	Commercial (adulterated)
linalool	1.2-1.8	1.9	3.4	2.0	0.4	0.8-1.9 same
citronellal	2.3	2.6	24.6	2.2	0.7	32-38 more
caryophyllene	2.7-3.6	1.0	11.7	4.3	9.5	0.3-0.8 less
neral	28.5-31	25.3	15.3	39.25	24.5	0.6-3.7 less
geranial	32-38	34.5	25.0	22.54	37.2	1.2-5.2 less
geranyl acetate	2.5-3.5	5.0	6.1	trace	0.5	13-18 more
nerol	1.6	0.5	0.4	4.1	0.1	0.4-1.3 same
geraniol	2.5-3	2.5	1.3	3.6	0.1	11-14 more
carophyllene oxide	3.6-7	3.0	2.1	0.6	2.5	0.04-0.08 less

The commercial oils differ from the natural oil mainly in containing significant amounts of citronellol and very much higher levels of citronellal with lower levels of neral and geranial. Additionally they also contain much higher levels of geraniol and geranyl acetate with extremely low levels of caryophyllene & caryophyllene oxide. The levels of linalool & nerol are comparable. [Perfumer & Flavourist (1985) Vol.10 No.6 pgs.30-2]
Safety application for melissa oil is undetermined at present.

Spanish oregano oil (Thymus capitatus) Labiatae
Both Spanish oregano and Spanish marjoram oils are obtained from species of thyme native to the Iberian peninsula comprising Spain and Portugal. The essential oil of Spanish oregano differs from that of garden thyme in having a higher content of carvacrol than thymol.
[Perfumer & Flavourist (1980) Vol.5 No.2 pgs.37]

Safety applications may be tentatively assumed to be comparable to that of garden thyme oil, red. **The recommended safe limit of use is at 8%.**

thyme oil, wild (Thymus serpyllum) Labiatae
Wild thyme is not cultivated and a limited quantity is collected from the wild for obtaining the essential oil by steam distillation. It is not as important as garden thyme, T. vulgaris but the oil is very occasionally found on the international market.

Composition: The total phenol content of thymol and carvacrol varies from 48 -78%. 0.1-15% borneol, 2.5-9.6% geraniol, 22-45% linalool & linalyl acetate, 0.4-5.2% bornyl acetate, 1.6-4% geranyl acetate and 0.7-6.5% 1,8-cineole. [Perfumer & Flavourist (1978) Vol.3 No.2 pgs.49]

Safety application for wild thyme oil may be tentatively assumed to be comparable to that of garden thyme oil, red based on their similarity. **The recommended safe limit of use is at 8%.**

yarrow oil (Achillea millefolium) Compositae
Yarrow is a common European herb growing wild throughout the temperate regions. Several species of Achillea form a complex grouping that is difficult to separate. Another species A. collina may also be used as yarrow in Eastern Europe. In North America, A. lanulosa and A. ptarmica are often also encountered as yarrow. The essential oil is steam distilled from the flowers, having a deep blue colour and characteristic aroma of chamomile and wormwood.

Composition: 9.4% a-pinene, 6% camphene, 7% b-pinene, 12.35% sabinene, 1.3% a-terpinene, 1.7% limonene, 9.6% 1,8-cineole, 3.7% g-terpinene, 3.7% p-cymene, 8.6% isoartemisia ketone, 1.4% allo-ocimene, 17.8% camphone, 2% bornyl acetate, 4.3% terpinen-4-ol, 1.6% caryophyllene, 2.55% borneol and an average content of 9.53% chamazulene.
[Perfumer & Flavourist (1984) Vol.9 No.4 pgs.43-8]

The chemical composition of yarrow oil most closely resembles that of the chamomiles and also of wormwood. Safety application can be tentatively assumed to be comparable to the chamomile oils. **The recommended safe limit of use is 4%.**

santolina oil (Santolina chamaecyparissus) Compositae

Santolina is related to both chamomile and yarrow and the essential oil, steam distilled from the flowers and leaves, possesses a fresh, camphoraceous, herbaceous and spicy aroma reminiscent of chamomile Roman and wormwood.

Composition: 2-5% b-pinene, 2-5% sabinene, 3.6-9.6% myrcene, 0.8-1.7% limonene, 8.6-18% b-phellandrene, 1.6% 1,8-cineole, 0.8-2.3% terpinolene, 8.5-34% artemisia ketone, 0.4-1.8% longipinene, 0.4-1.2% artemisia alcohol, 1.3-2.6% camphone, 1.7-2.2% g-curcumene, 0.8-1% borneol, 0.4-2.7% germacrene D, 0.7-1.5% bicyclo-germacrene, 0.8-1.7% ar-curcumene and 9-17.4% longiverbenone. [Perfumer & Flavourist (1992) Vol.17 No.6 pgs.53-6]

Safety application for santolina oil can be tentatively assumed to be comparable to that of wormwood oil based on the resemblance of their chemical composition. **The recommended safe limit of use is 2%.**

balsamite oil (Chrysanthemum balsamita) Compositae

Balsamite is among the composite plants possessing insecticidal properties. The essential oil is not very common, but is highly valued by some perfumers as a fragrance ingredient. The insecticidal action of the balsamite oil is particularly active against aphids. This action is due to the oil's content of pyrethrin I. Balsamite resembles tansy in existing as several chemical races producing essential oils of different chemical composition.

Composition: 2.6% limonene, 0.6% 1,8-cineole, 0.8% a-thujone, 51.5% carvone, 0.46% bornyl acetate, 4.7% cubebene, 0.5% zingiberene and pyrethrin I.

The pyrethrin I was unequivocally characterised as a constituent of the leaves.
[Perfumer & Flavourist (1977) Vol.2 No.2 pgs.29 & (1986) Vol.11 No.1 pgs.29 & (1987) Vol.12 No.1 pgs.35]
Safety application for balsamite oil is undetermined at present.

zdravetz oil (Geranium macrorrhizum) Geraniaceae

Zdravetz oil is water or steam distilled from the European cranesbill (Geranium macrorrhizum) plant of the Geraniaceae family. It is much less important than geranium oil steam distilled from South African Perlagonium species, also of the same Geraniaceae family. Zdravetz oil has been produced for over 50 years in Bulgaria. Some zdravetz oil is also produced in Yugoslavia. The major component of the oil, germacrone has a tendency to crystallise causing the oil to become a semi-crystalline material at normal room temperature.

Composition: 50% germacrone, with 14% terpenes including a-pinene, d-3-carene, a-phellandrene, limonene, g-terpinene, terpinolene, p-cymene, b-elemene, caryophyllene, g-murolene, a-humulene, ar-curcumene, d-cadinene, calamenene and a-santalene; and 20% alcohols including b-eudesmol, junenol and elemol.
[Perfumer & Flavourist (1978) Vol.3 No.2 pgs.49 & (1980) Vol.5 No.4 pgs.35]
Safety application for zdravetz oil is undetermined at present.

valerian oil (Valeriana officinalis) Valerianaceae

Valerian is a European plant that can be found widely distributed throughout the Serbian region of Yugoslavia and is grown as an ornamental. The essential oil is obtained by steam distillation of the dried comminuted roots, produced in Belgium, France, Hungary and Russia. Valerian oil is primarily used in flavourings and pharmaceuticals with a limited quantity in fragrances, particularly in Europe.

Composition: principal constituents - 2-12% elemol, 0-18% valeranone, 3.3-16% valerenal, with 4-10% a-pinene, 8-14.4% camphene, 1% b-pinene, 1.5-11% limonene, b-terpinene & 1,8-cineole, 0.4-3.2% caryophyllene, 0.6-6% a-gurjunene, 0.7-2.6% allo-aromadendrene, 0.3-1.7% germacrene D, 1.5-7.2% bicyclo-elemene, 1-3.4% bornyl acetate and 1.2-3% b-elemene.

The essential oil was found to contribute to the pharmacological activity of valerian root. Valerian oil is used in the pharmaceutical industry for its calming and spasmolytic properties. The most active compounds were found in the oxygenated fraction. Valerenal possessed central nervous system depressant activity and with valerenic acid was pharmacologically active at low doses. [Perfumer & Flavourist (1985) Vol.10 No.5 pgs.98-102 & (1987) Vol.12 No.1 pgs.52]

Safety application for valerian oil is undetermined at present.

parsnip root oil (Pastinaca sativa) Umbelliferae

The parsnip is related to the carrot and both are used in a similar way as root vegetables. However the composition of their essential oils varies considerably.

Composition: 40-70% terpinolene, 17-40% myristicin, with 14 other monoterpenes and 2 sesquiterpenes. [Perfumer & Flavourist (1976) Vol.1 No.2 pgs.20]

Safety application for parsnip root oil is undetermined at present.

chervil oil (Anthriscus cerefolium) Umbelliferae

Chervil is cultivated mainly in the low countries such as the Netherlands and Belgium. The essential oil obtained by steam distillation of the herb is extremely rare.

Composition: 75% methyl chavicol, 22.3% 1-allyl-2,4-dimenthoxybenzene (osmorhizole), with b-pinene and b-phellandrene. [Perfumer & Flavourist (1983) Vol.8 No.3 pgs.72-3]

The methyl chavicol (estragole) content of chervil oil is intermediate between tarragon oil and basil oil. Safety application for chervil oil may be tentatively assumed to be comparable to both the other essential oils. **Recommended limit of use at 4%**

opoponax absolute (Opoponax chironium) Umbelliferae

Until additional work is completed, the IFRA recommends that only opoponax absolute which is obtained by alcoholic extraction should be used, and not the crude opoponax gum. This recommendation is based on unpublished RIFM findings communicated privately to the IFRA, that alcohol-extracted opoponax absolute did not show any sensitising potential.

storax resinoid (Styrax officinalis) Styracaceae

The IFRA recommends that crude storax resinoid should not be used as a fragrance ingredient. Only storax resinoid produced by neutralising with aqueous alkali followed by solvent extraction should be used. This recommendation is based on unpublished RIFM findings communicated privately to the IFRA, that crude storax resinoid showed sensitising potential.

mustard oil (Brassica nigra) Cruciferae
The United States NIOSH determined the oral toxicity of mustard oil to be 0.148g/kg (rat)

Mustard oil is distilled from black mustard seeds after expression of the fixed oil and maceration in tepid water to allow interaction between the glycoside sinigrin and the enzyme myrosin. It is an intensely pungent, irritating, colourless to pale yellow liquid containing not less than 92% allyl isothiocyanate.

Mustard oil is an extremely powerful irritant and vesicant. When applied undiluted it causes rapid blistering of the skin. **It should not be inhaled or tasted undiluted.**
[Martindale Extra-Pharmacopoeia 28th ed. 1982]

Allyl isothiocyanate is a phytochemical paradox with a very complex nature. This compound is toxic, a strong lachrimator (tear producing as in tear gas), skin vesicant and recommended by the IFRA not to be used in fragrances; but at the same time is also considered as GRAS (generally recognised as safe) by the FEMA, is used as a food flavour and appears to have a strong anti-carcinogenic potential. The U. S. National Cancer Institute considers it among a class of 14 plant substances offering significant hope in preventing the development of cancer in humans and animals. It is found in numerous food plants and is consumed as a vegetable in relatively large amounts in the diet of humans and animals. Of all the isothiocyanates found in nature, allyl isothiocyanate is the only one accepted as having a GRAS status by the FEMA.
[Perfumer & Flavourist (1992) Vol.17 No.5 pgs.107-9]

horseradish oil (Amoracia rusticana) Cruciferae
Horseradish oil has some economic importance but is not a terribly important essential oil. Composition: 44.3-55.7% allyl isothiocyanate, 38.4-51.3% 2-phenylethyl isothiocyanate, 1.6-2.5% allyl thiocyanate, 0.6-4% 4-pentenyl isothiocyanate, 0.35-2.7% 2-butyl isothiocyanate.
[Perfumer & flavourist (1981) Vol.6 No.1 pgs.45-6]

The compound allyl isothiocyanate, found in substantial amounts in both mustard oil and horseradish oil has an odour and taste reminiscent of mustard and horseradish combined. The pure compound is so strong that no accompanying constituents' taste or odour is noted and is always used in very low concentration for this reason.

95% of the world's consumption of allyl isothiocyanate is used in food flavouring with only 5% being used in negative perfumery for repelling odours. Negative odours are used in household products to induce a repelling odour and taste to prevent young children from drinking otherwise pleasant smelling products like cleaning fluids, glues, paints, eraser ink, etc.
[Perfumer & Flavourist (1992) Vol.17 No.5 pgs.107-9]

Considering its nature, mustard oil is clearly not suitable for aromatherapy and is recommended not to be used for this purpose. Although having a lower content of allyl isothiocyanate, the situation of horseradish oil is comparable to that of mustard oil and is also recommended not to be used in aromatherapy.

wintergreen oil (Gaultheria procumbens) Ericaceae

Wintergreen (also called checkerberry) is an aromatic evergreen creeper not exceeding 6in in height, native to eastern North America. It is found in cool damp woods in the shade of other evergreen shrubs and trees particularly rhododendrons and mountain laurels, growing prolifically in the vicinity of the Appalachian Mountains from Georgia in the south to Canada. During the summer months, when the leaves yield the highest quantity of oil, they are picked and like sweet birch bark, steeped in warm water before distilling. Wintergreen like sweet birch contains a glycoside which requires an aqueous enzymatic action to liberate the essential oil. The leaves of wintergreen contain the highest amount of the glycoside, monotropitin (formerly gaultherin). Wintergreen oil has been produced in the United States since the early 17th century, but is always a small volume item. [Perfumer & Flavourist (1979) Vol.3 No.6 pgs.32-3]

In addition to a limited use in perfumery for fern and cypress-type fragrances, wintergreen has also been used in pharmaceutical preparations in particular for reducing the swelling of tissues. Wintergreen tea was formerly used in the treatment of rheumatism, dysentery, delayed menstruation. [Krochmal & Krochmal 1972]

Both wintergreen oil and sweet birch oil contain a comparably high content of methyl salicylate, at up to 98%. However the United States NIOSH determined the oral toxicity of wintergreen oil in rats to be 0.887g/kg. This is twice as toxic as sweet birch oil with an oral toxicity value at 1.7g/kg. Additional oral toxic doses were also determined at 11g/kg for mice; at 1g/kg for guineapigs; at 1.3g/kg for rabbits; at 0.17g/kg for hamsters and at 2.1g/kg for dogs.

It is absorbed through the skin and is applied undiluted or in liniments and ointments for the relief of pain in lumbago, sciatica and rheumatism. [Martindale's Extra-Pharmacopoeia 28th ed. 1982]

Methyl salicylate tested at 8% for 48 hours on 27 volunteers, did not produce any irritation or sensitisation reactions. Incorporated into most topically applied pain relievers, methyl salicylate has been evaluated as a moderate irritant at a concentration as low as 1%.

Sensitivity to methyl salicylate have been reported in 2 patients confirmed by patch tests.
[J.K. Morgan, Br J clin Pract (1968) 22, 261]

Urticaria and angioneurotic oedema occurred on several occasions in a patient sensitive to aspirin following exposure to liniments, toothpaste and candy containing methyl salicylate.
[F. Speer, Ann allergy (1979) 43, 36]

Ingestion of relatively small amounts of methyl salicylate may cause severe poisoning and death. Signs of poisoning include nausea, vomiting, acidosis, pulmonary oedema, pneumonia and convulsions. The lethal dose for children is calculated as 4 - 8ml. Signs common to all such poisonings being excitation of the central nervous system, abnormally rapid breathing, fever, high blood pressure and increased heartbeat, generalized convulsions and coma. Death results from respiratory failure after a period of unconsciousness. A 10-year old boy suffered from severe metabolic acidosis after ingesting approximately 10ml of methyl salicylate. Many cases of methyl salicylate poisoning have been reported with a 50-60% death rate.

The NIOSH determined the oral toxic dose of wintergreen oil in humans to be 0.17g/kg.
Accidental ingestion of 1-3 oz. of wintergreen oil by patients showing myocardial failure resulted in 21% of the ingested amount still circulating in the blood after 1.5hr. The methyl salicylate is hydrolysed to salicylic acid to a considerable extent in the intestines with some residue appearing in the urine. Lethal concentrations of total circulating plasma salicylate in humans were 2-3 times higher than those in dogs at the time of death, due to a lack of adequate detoxification mechanisms in humans. The level of total plasma salicylate resulting in death was lower in female dogs because of their higher fat content, than in male dogs.

It was reported that a significantly greater percentage of women delivering defective babies had taken a salicylate preparation during the first trimester of pregnancy than had women delivering normal babies, possibly related to methyl salicylate's metabolism to salicylic acid.

Two seamen suffered acute poisoning after drinking wintergreen oil. One of them drank 30ml and survived while the other drank 90ml and died. [J.J. Canselmo, J Am med Ass (1948) 136, 651]

Twenty four hours after swallowing about 5ml of wintergreen oil, a 20 month old child was in a critical condition with poor chances of survival with a blood salicylate concentration of 727 mg per ml. He only survived following an exchange blood transfusion (reducing the blood salicylate concentration by 59%) and intravenous fluids.
[J.T. Adams, J Am med Ass (1957) 165, 1563]

Wintergreen oil is too potent and hazardous to be suitable for use in aromatherapy.

---

savin oil (Juniperus sabina) Cupressaceae
Savin leaf oil is not very popular but finds some use in the compounding of pine fragrances. Composition: 2.2-6.8% a-pinene, 26-30% sabinene, 4% myrcene, 1.6-2.7% limonene, 0.6-1.2% 1,8-cineole, 1.7% methyl citronellate, 2-3.2% terpinen-4-ol, 37.5-38% sabinyl acetate, 1% sabinol, 0.8-1.8% citronellol, 1.5-4.5% a-cadinene.
[Perfumer & Flavourist (1982) Vol.7 No.4 pgs.46-9]

Savin oil used as an emmenagogue may cause haematuria and violent gastrointestinal irritation in addition to pelvic congestion. Serious and fatal cases of poisoning have resulted from its use as a supposed abortifacient. It is a violent irritant both externally and internally.
[Martindale Extra-Pharmacopoeia 28th ed. 1982]

Savin oil has an irritant effect on the digestive mucosa, causing congestion of the kidneys with haematuria, congestion of other abdominal organs, menorrhagia and abortion. Toxic effects are due to sabinene, sabinol and sabinyl acetate having similar effects to the thujane, thujol and thujone of thuja leaf oil. [17th Eurotox Meeting (1964) Brussels]

The IFRA recommendation is not to use essential oils with a sabinol content above 3% as a fragrance ingredient and that savin oil should not be used. [IFRA Report 1980]
This recommendation is based on the high toxicity of savin oil due to its sabinol content of 35-55%. [Gosselin, Hodge, Smith & Gleason (1976) Clinical Toxicology of Commercial Products]

Savin oil is sufficiently toxic to be considered too hazardous for normal use. It is therefore unnecessary for irritation, sensitisation or phototoxicity tests to be conducted as the results would only be academic. **The recommendation for savin oil is that it should not be used.**

lily-of-the-valley oil (Convallaria majalis) Liliaceae
Composition: a-phellandrene, a-terpinene, limonene, linalool oxide, 2,2,6-trimethyl-6-vinyl-tetrahydrofuran, hexen-1-ol, linalool, citronellol, phenyl ethyl alcohol, hydrocinnamyl alcohol, neral, geranial, cirtonellal, benzaldehyde, geranyl acetate, neryl acetate, benzyl acetate, phenyl ethyl acetate, phenyl propyl acetate, benzyl carpoate, cinnamyl carpoate, methyl anthranilate, methyl salicylate, 3-hexenyl acetate, benzyl cynide, indole and cresodolin. **No quantitative data was available.** [Perfumer & Flavourist (1978) Vol.3 No.1 pgs.56]

Lily-of-the-valley is a plant with small white flowers probably originating from Asia and is now found in the wild state throughout Europe. When the flowers dry out, they lose part of the ethereal green-floral note but retain a musky sweetness with a light green note, for weeks if enclosed in a plastic envelope. In contrast, lilac blossoms lose all odour and change to a rusty colour when wilting. This unique floral characteristic of lily-of-the-valley is of distinct interest to the creative perfumer and is important in perfumery having a universal application.

The fragrance of lily-of-the-valley flowers is appreciated by almost everyone, but it is extremely difficult to obtain the essential oil by steam distillation, and the natural flower oil is not commercially available. Flower stalks are collected from the humid woods of southern France and first extracted with pentane twice and then the extract distilled in vacuum. The essential oil consists of about 70% citronellol, nerol, geraniol, and their acetates.

Attempts have been made to obtain the concrete and absolute of lily-of-the-valley with petroleum ether extraction, but these extraction products are only used for scientific research. Most of the commercial products with a lily-of-the-valley fragrance are formulated with synthetic compounds fixed with olibanum, storax resinoid and Tolu Balsam. It is offered as a straight perfume oil known as muguet. Some lily-of-the-valley compositions also contain lilac compounds. In general the lily-of-the-valley scent is compatible with many floral notes.

The lily-of-the-valley scent is incorporated into numerous luxury perfumes including Quelques Fleur, Arpege, Je Reviens, Replique, Chantilly, l'Air du Temps, Intimate, Diorissimo, Fidgi, Madam Rochas, Rive Gauche and Aliage. In Premiere, lily-of-the-valley is blended with gardenia and honeysuckle and in Armani, with jasmine, neroli and hyacinth.
[Perfumer & Flavourist (1980) Vol.5 No.6 pgs.1-8 & (1986) Vol.11 No.6 pgs31-6]

lilac oil (Syringa vulgaris) Oleaceae
Composition: a-pinene, ocimene, methyl benzyl ether, hydroquinone dimethyl ether, lilac alcohol (4 stereoisomers), cis-3-hexenol, linalool, benzaldehyde, anisaldehyde, cresol, cresyl acetate, cis-3-hexenyl acetate and several sesquiterpenes. **No quantitative data was available**
[Perfumer & Flavourist (1978) Vol.3 No.2 pgs.46]

The lilac is a spring flowering shrub, probably originating in Iran and introduced to Spain in the 16th century. Although the blossoms have a most pleasing scent, the essential oil is of little commercial importance because when recovered from the flowers, the oil only retains poor or non-lilac odour qualities. Among the few commercially available natural lilac products is the absolute from Bulgaria. The essential oil is extremely difficult to produce because of destruction of the scent by the distillation process. Nevertheless, the lilac odour has for a long time appealed to the creative instincts of the perfumer.

The most important fragrant components of lilac oil are the 4 stereoisomers of lilac alcohol (b,5-dimethyl-5-vinyl-2-tetra-hydrofuran ethanol) which amounts to 70% of the essential oil. Many other components have been identified in lilac oil but not quantified.

Lilac tends to be less delicate than lily-of-the-valley and not as distinctive as rose. Single floral fragrances of lilac are only of minor importance. The most valuable application for lilac has been in the numerous fragrance formulations where the lilac odour can be used to support another floral theme. Fragrances where it has been incorporated as part of the floral composition includes Quelques Fleur by Houbigant; Arpege by Lanvin; Fidgi by Guy Laroche; Fleurs de Rocaille by Caron; Sortilege by Pier Auge and Chant d'Aromes by Guerlain.
[Perfumer & Flavourist (1979) Vol.4 No.5 pgs.1-4]

gardenia oil (Gardenia jasminoides) Rubiaceae

Gardenias are found mainly in the Far East, growing particularly well together with osmanthus and tuberose in the Chunking region of China. They are also widely distributed in Japan. At the turn of the century, gardenia was cultivated in Reunion Island for the perfumery. As in the case of other delicate flowers, steam distillation of gardenia flowers gives very poor results. Enfleurage and solvent extraction are more successful, producing the absolute. Gardenia and carnation are considered to be balanced floral components with lavender.

Composition: benzyl acetate, linalool, linalyl acetate, methyl anthranilate, styrallyl acetate and terpineol. **No quantitative data was available**. The absolute also contained beta ocimene, methyl benzoate, hexyl tiglate, cis-3-hexenol, cis-3-hexenyl tiglate and cis-3-hexenyl benzoate. Benzyl acetate was present in the largest amount but styrallyl acetate was the most suggestive of the gardenia scent.

The natural gardenia oil is very scarcely produced and synthetic compounds fixed with labdanum, myrrh and Tolu balsam are more often used to create the gardenia odour in perfumery. Gardenia is considered a secondary floral in perfumery but is important in the role of fragrance modifier remaining a valuable floral-green note. It is included in many established perfumes including Aphrodisia, l'Air du Temps, Vent Vert, Cabochard, Detchema, Caleche, Aliage, Michelle, Tatiana and Premiere. [Perfumer & Flavourist (1983) Vol.8 No.5 pgs.31-7]

mignonette oil (Reseda odorata) Resedaceae

Mignonette originated in Asia Minor and at the turn of the century it was used to produce a natural flower oil with a vibrant green-floral odour used in high class perfumes.

Steam distillation of the flowers yielded a very low yield of 0.002% of essential oil. Solvent extraction resulting in a concrete and absolute produced a higher yield ranging from 0.07 - 0.15%. In the early part of this century, up to 40 metric tons of mignonette flowers were processed for perfumery, but by the middle of the century, production had almost completely ceased. Natural mignonette oil have not been available for quite a number of years. The chemical composition of mignonette flower oil is not well known. Almost all mignonette fragrances are synthetically formulated with compounds possessing similar odours.
[Perfumer & Flavourist (1990) Vol.15 No.6 pgs.18-21]

carnation oil (Dianthus caryophyllus) Caryophyllaceae

The carnation is found mostly in dry sunny places in the Mediterranean region. The carnation flowers yield 0.05% of essential oil which is important for using in fine fragrances because of its rich clove-like aroma. The absolute achieved a limited use in the fragrance industry having a sweet, heavy, honey-like aroma reminiscent of clove. Although carnation oil was rarely used, it was a very useful perfume base.

Composition: 40% benzyl benzoate, 30% eugenol, 7% phenyl ethyl alcohol, 5% benzyl salicylate and 1% methyl salicylate. The phenolic content of carnation oil is probably responsible for its antimicrobial action and it has been used as a room disinfectant and anti-moulding agent in syrups. [Perfumer & Flavourist (1985) Vol.10 No.1 pgs44-8]

cassie oil (Acacia farnesiana) Leguminosae

Cassie is a small tree up to 3m in height bearing small yellow flowers arranged in the shape of a ball. Growing wild in Africa, Australia, western India and southern China, it has long been cultivated in the Mediterranean countries. The flower extracts are used in fine fragrances. The concrete is produced in southern France, and on treatment with alcohol, yielded the absolute. Steam distillation of the concrete yields an essential oil which is only used for scientific research and is not commercially available. French production has declined in recent years and presently cassie is cultivated for perfumery in the north African countries of Egypt, Algeria and Morocco, as well as in South Africa. [Perfumer & Flavourist (1987) Vol.12 No.6 pgs.31-6]

Cassie oil is extracted from the flowers and possesses a warm, powdery, herbaceous, floral (violet) top note with a tenacious balsamic base note. It is a very interesting raw material used primarily for fragrance formulation and to a limited extent for flavour formulation as well.
Composition: 18.5% methyl salicylate, 13.5% farnesol, 11.8% geraniol, 8.2% o-cresol, 4.7% b-ionone, 1.26% a-terpineol and 1% linalool. [Perfumer & Flavourist (1984) Vol.9 No.3 pgs.35-6]

The flowers of another species of Acacia, A. romaine/cavinea produce roman cassie oil with a different composition: 8.7% linalool, 8.4% geraniol, 7.4% benzaldehyde, 7.2% citronellol, 6.6% a-terpineol, 5.5% methyl salicylate, 5.3% a-pinene, 5.2% benzoic alcohol, 4.8% limonene, 4.3% camphene, 4.1% geranyl acetate, 3.4% p-cymene, 3.1% b-pinene, 1.3% methyl eugenol, 1.2% o-cresol and 1.1% m-cresol. [Perfumer & Flavourist (1982) Vol.7 No.1 pgs.45]

licorice oil (Glycyrrhiza glabra) Leguminosae

Licorice is a perennial subshrub with long horizontal underground stems. Since early times, licorice root has been used in traditional medicine and in the preparation of confections and beverages. The active principle of this plant is a triterpene glycoside, glycyrrhizin which is responsible for its sweet taste. It is pharmacologically and commercially important as a solid extract prepared from the roots by hot water extraction followed by final drying into sticks. The essential oil is much less commonly encountered, the aroma being due not to any one single compound but to a diverse mixture of constituents.

Composition: the main constituents are acetol, propionic acid, 2-acetylfuran, 2-acetyl-pyrrole and furfuryl alcohol; with pentanol, hexanol, trans-3-hexanol, 1-oct-en-3-ol, linalool oxide A, linalool oxide B, tetramethyl pyrazine, terpinen-4-ol, a-terpineol, benzaldehyde, benzyl alcohol, phenyl ethyl alcohol and geraniol. [Perfumer & Flavourist (1986) Vol.11 No.6 pgs.44-5]

Safety application for licorice oil is undetermined at present.

blackcurrant bud oil (Ribes nigrum) Rosaceae

The blackcurrant bush is grown extensively in central and northern Europe for its berries, which are generally used in jellies and as flavours for ice-creams, yoghurts and alcoholic beverages. In some regions, especially Burgundy, the bushes are pruned during winter and the cuttings already containing the hibernating buds are prepared as an alcoholic tincture and used to enhance the flavour of the juice, especially after the juice has been stored for a few months.

A portion of the buds are used for obtaining the absolute, which serves as a flavour enhancer like the tincture but it is also used as a fragrance ingredient. The absolute is a dark-green paste having a very characteristic, penetrating and powerful odour. An essential oil is obtained by steam distillation of the absolute, yielding about 12-15%. It is a pale coloured liquid having the typical powerful odour of the absolute. [Perfumer & Flavourist (1985) Vol.9 No.6 pgs.39-42]

The bud of the common blackcurrant plant possesses a strong characteristic aroma and extracts prepared from it have been used in fragrance formulations. The extract is commercially known as 'bourgeons de cassissier'. It is most commonly encountered as either an absolute or a concrete, but the essential oil is also available. [Perfumer & Flavourist (1987) Vol.12 No.5 pgs.55-8]

Composition: 1% a-thujene, 1.3-9% a-pinene, 1.2% camphene, 1.8-69% sabinene, 1-10% b-pinene, 3% myrcene, 1% a-phellandrene, 2.8-46% d-3-carene, 1% a-terpinene, 11-14% limonene, 2-25% b-phellendrene, 5% b-ocimene, 1% g-terpinene, 9-20% terpinolene, 2.4-4% terpinen-4-ol, 1% bornyl acetate, 1.2-5% b-caryophyllene, 1% a-humulene, 1.4% spathulenol, 1.2% caryophyllene oxide, 0.75% germacrene D, 0.6% germacrene B.

The typical and potent odour of blackcurrant oil is not due to the monoterpenes but the sesquiterpenes content and also to the presence of sulphur compounds at 0.08-0.15%.
[Perfumer & Flavourist (1991) Vol.16 No.6 pgs.49]

Safety application for blackcurrant bud oil is undetermined at present. However the composition does not suggest any probable hazardous components.

Asia (India, China & Japan) -

olibanum oil (Boswellia carterii) Burseraceae

Olibanum is a natural oleo-gum-resin exudate which is harvested in the form of tears or lumps from trees growing mainly in Aden and Eritrea. Some olibanum is also found in Saudi Arabia and northwestern India. Olibanum oil is obtained by steam distillation of the exudate. It is of interest in perfumery because of its unique odour characteristics which make it a valuable ingredient for fine fragrance compounding and for its fixative properties. An absolute is also available. [Perfumer & Flavourist (1982) Vol.7 No.1 pgs.48-50]

Composition: 1.4% a-thujene, 3.5% a-pinene, 1.7% limonene, 1.6% 1,8-cineole, 1.3% b-ocimene, 12.7% octanol, 2% linalool, 60% octyl acetate, 1% bornyl acetate, 1.8% isocembrene, 1.4% cembrene and 2.7% incensol. [Perfumer & Flavourist (1992) Vol.17 No.3 pgs.61-6]

The RIFM conducted safety testing only for olibanum gum and absolute. Until safety information becomes available for olibanum oil, its safety application may be assumed to be comparable to that of the other 2 products. **The recommended safe limit of use is at 8%.**

galangal (Alpinia galanga) Zingiberaceae

Galangal is a tropical plant related to ginger, cardamon and turmeric, native to India and Malaysia. It is used to produce an essential oil in limited quantities.

Composition: 7-10% a-pinene, 6.2% a-thujene, 1.6-11.5% b-pinene, 5.5-47.3% 1,8-cineole, 1.6-4.3% limonene, 0.7-1.4% myrcene, 1-2% g-terpinene, 1% terpinolene, 0.2-4.7% a-terpineol, 0.3-6% terpinen-4-ol, 0.4-2.5% bornyl acetate, 1.8-5% geranyl acetate, 1.6% citronellyl acetate, 1.5% eugenyl acetate, 1% chavicyl acetate, 10.7% bergamotene, 18.2% trans-b-farnesene, 2% ar-curcumene, 16.2% b-bisabolene, 2% pentadecane, 1.6% b-sesqui-phellandrene and 2.5% caryophyllene oxide. [Perfumer & Flavourist (1986) Vol.11 No.1 pgs.31-3]

Safety application for galangal oil is tentatively assumed to be comparable to that of the other 3 Zingeriberaceae plants. **The recommended safe limit of use is at 4%.**

agarwood oil (Aquilaria agallocha) Thymelaceae

The agarwood is a softwood tree found in evergreen forests particularly in the hilly regions from India to Burma and Vietnam. Trees attaining an age of about 80 years are reported to possess the highest yield of oil, about 7-9 kg. Irregular patches of dark streaks and blotches of oleoresin are impregnated in the wood and are particularly odoriferous. The usual method of obtaining agarwood oil is by water distillation. The wood is first chipped and soaked in water for 4-5 days. The chips are then ground into small pieces, which are further soaked in water for another 2 days before distilling. The essential oil possesses a characteristic balsamic aroma with a sandalwood-like tonality.

Composition: a-agarofuran, 0.6% b-agarofuran, dihydro-b-agarofuran, isodihydro-a-agarofuran, 0.6% nor-ketoagarofuran, 4.7% agarospirol, agarol, jinkohol, 2.4% jinkohol II, 4% jinkohol-eremol, 2.9% kusunol, karanone, 2.4% dihydro karanone, oxo-agarospirol, iso-agarospirol and gmelofuran. [Perfumer & Flavourist (1985) Vol.10 No.3 pgs.27-30]

Safety application for agarwood oil is tentatively assumed to be comparable to that of sandalwood oil. **The recommended safe limit of use is at 10%**

spikenard oil (Nardostachys jatamansi) Valerianaceae

Spikenard is an erect perennial growing at an elevation of 3-5000m in the Himalayan regions of India. The roots are used to produce an essential oil in limited quantities in the Kanpur-Kananuj region. Spikenard is also valued as a medicinal plant in India and the roots are sold in the marketplace in many villages in the northern states. Another species, the Chinese spikenard (Nardostachys chinensis) is an ancient medicinal plant in China. An essential oil can also be obtained from Chinese spikenard, but very little of it is available commercially, so is of minor interest. Spikenard oil has similar odour qualities with valerian oil and also patchouli oil. although it is slightly more earthy than patchouli oil.

Composition of **Chinese spikenard oil** - 8% aristole-1-ol, 2% 9,10-aristolene, 8.6% 1,10-aristolene, 32.8% b-maliene and 13% 1,2,9,10-tetradehydro-aristolane.

Composition of **Indian spikenard oil** - 30% b-gurjunene, 30% z-patchoulene, 1.7% seychellene, 1.4% b-ionone, 6% patchoulol, 6.2% hydroxy aristolenone with aristolenone, b-patchoulene and a-gurjunene. [Perfumer & Flavourist (1986) Vol.10 No.6 pgs.32-8]

Safety application for spikenard oil is tentatively assumed to be similar to that of patchouli oil. **The recommended limit of use is 10%**

tejpat oil (Cinnamomum tamala) Lauraceae

Tejpat is the Indian cinnamon, although not as important as Sri Lankan cinnamon. The leaves have been used to produce an essential oil similar to Sri Lankan cinnamon leaf oil.

Composition: 1.5% a-pinene, 1% 1,8-cineole, 3.2% p-cymene, 1.2% eugenyl acetate and 78% eugenol. [Perfumer & Flavourist (1983) Vol.8 No.3 pgs.74]

Safety application for Indian cinnamon leaf oil is tentatively assumed to be comparable to Sri Lankan cinnamon leaf oil. **The recommended safe limit of use is at 10%.**

vateria oil (Vateria indica) Dipterocarpaceae

The vateria tree is distributed in the forests on the western mountain slopes of India at elevations up to 1200m. The tree produces an oleoresin important in the traditional medicine of India for treating ulcers and carbuncles. Water and steam distillation of the oleoresin yields 1.5% of a yellowish brown essential oil.

Composition: 11.5% d-camphene, 25% a-pinene, 6% b-pinene, 19% limonene, 1% chamazulene, 10% b-caryophyllene, 4% d-camphor, 6.5% a-terpineol, 10% d-borneol and 7% thymol. [Perfumer & Flavourist (1982) Vol.7 No.4 pgs.15-7]

Safety applications for vateria oil is undetermined at present.

skimmia oil (Skimmia laureola) Rutaceae

Skimmia is an evergreen shrub growing wild in the medium to high elevations in the western Himalayas, especially in the middle and inner Himalayan ranges over a wide area of Uttar Pradesh province of India. The essential oil obtained from the leaves possesses an odour that is quite similar to petitgrain bigarade oil.

Composition: 51-67.4% linalyl acetate, 18.4-27% linalool with a-pinene, b-phellendrene, neral, geranial, methyl heptenone, geraniol, camphene, furfural, chamazulene, guaiazulene, vanillin, bergaptene and isopimpinellin. [Perfumer & Flavourist (1982) Vol.7 No.2 pgs.38-9]

Safety application for skimmia oil is undetermined at present.

abutilon oil (Abutilon indicum) Malvaceae

Abutilon is an aromatic annual herb commonly found in the Madhya Pradesh province of India. Steam distillation of the flowering tops yields 0.15% of a reddish-brown essential oil.

Composition: 0.1% a-pinene, 1% 1,8-cineole, 11.6% caryophyllene, 0.6% borneol, 13% geraniol, 2% geranyl acetate, 2% caryophyllene oxide, 0.5% elemene, 22% eudesmol and 2.8% farnesol. [Perfumer & Flavourist (1983) Vol.5 No.3 pgs.39]

Safety application for abutilon oil is undetermined at present.

asafoetida oil (Ferula asafoetida) Umbelliferae

Asafoetida is an umbelliferous plant native to India and the Middle Eastern countries. The essential oil distilled from the seeds is light yellow in colour, having a very pungent, lingering, sulphuroceous odour with a very warm, sweet, balsamic undertone.

Composition: 1.7-2.3% a-pinene, 1% camphene, 2-2.5% myrcene, 0.6% limonene, 4.6-6% longifolene, 3.8-5% caryophyllene, 15.2-17.2% b-selinene, 4.7-5% eugenol, 2.25-4.5% bornyl acetate, 1.5-2.4% fenchone, and 39% of a mixture of sesquiterpenes and 7.5% of a mixture of coumarins. The perculiar sulphuraceous odour is due to the presence of sulphur compounds - 35% 2-butyl propenyl disulphide, 2-butyl 3-methyl thioallyl disulphide, and 1-methyl thiopropyl 1-propenyl disulphide. [Perfumer & Flavourist (1981) Vol.6 No.1 pgs.38]

Safety application for asafoetida oil is undetermined at present.

ammoniac gum oil (Dorema ammoniacum) Umbelliferae

Ammoniac is an umbelliferous perennial herb native to Iran, Afghanistan, Pakistan and India. The stem exudes a gum containing approximately 3% of essential oil possessing an odour that is somewhat sulphuraceous and musky.

Composition: 4% a-pinene, 0.8% b-pinene, 19.6% a-ferulene, 1.2% linalyl acetate, 38.6% citronellyl acetate, 4.2% doremone, 12.7% doremyl alcohol and 15% of a mixture of coumarins. [Perfurmer & Flavourist (1981) Vol.6 No.5 pgs.27]

Safety application for ammoniac gum oil is undetermined at present.

ajowan oil (Trachyspermum ammi) Umbelliferae
Ajowan is an umbelliferous plant native to India and Pakistan which are the principal sources of the essential oil, although the plant is also cultivated in Afghanistan, Iran and Egypt. The seeds are exported from India to Europe and North America to distill the essential oil.

Composition: 0.3-1.8% a-pinene, 0.5% camphene, 1.2-3.5% b-pinene, 0.3% myrcene, 0.4-0.8% d-3-carene, 0.2-5% limonene, 19-35% g-terpinene, 20.8-24% p-cymene, 45.2-48.5% thymol and 4.5-6.8% carvacrol. [Perfumer & Flavourist (1979) Vol.4 No.2 pgs.53]
The thymol and carvacrol content of ajowan oil is very similar to that of garden thyme oil, red. Safety application for ajowan oil may be tentatively assumed to be comparable to garden thyme oil, red. **Recommended limit of use at 8%**

blumea oil (Blumea mollis) Compositae
Blumea species are distributed in China, India, Australia, the Pacific region and S. Africa; Blumea mollis is found in the Malwa region near Ujain in India. Steam distilling the fresh flowering plant yields 0.034% of a dark brownish essential oil.

Composition: about 40% of monoterpenes with 60% of long chain aliphatic hydrocarbons including: 2,3-dimethoxy-p-cymene, 2,4,5-trimethoxy allylbenzene, caryophyllene oxide and 2-methyl-5-isopropyl cyclopentene. **No quantitative data was available.**
[Perfumer & Flavourist (1982) Vol.7 No.1 pgs.27-9]
Safety application for blumea oil is undetermined at present.

actractylis oil (Actractylodes lancea) Compositae
Actractylis is a plant native to China that has been used for a long time in traditional Chinese medicine. The essential oil is obtained by steam distilling the dried rhizome possessing a heavy, peppery, earthy and warm aroma. An absolute is also available, extracted with both petroleum ether and benzene.

Composition: b-eudesmol (main constituent), b-selinene, a-bisabolol, hinesol, elemol, furfurol, atractylodin and atractylodin. [Perfumer & Flavourist (1983) Vol.8 No.5 pgs.19]
Safety application for actractylis oil is undetermined at present.

magnolia oil (Magnolia grandiflora) Magnoliaceae
The magnolia tree originated in China, and was introduced into southern France and Italy at the end of the 18th century. Solvent extraction of the flowers yield a greenish-yellow concrete and steam distillation of the concrete yields the essential oil which is a semi-solid having the characteristic odour of magnolia flowers. The chemical composition of magnolia flower oil is not well known. The leaves of Italian magnolia have also been steam distilled to yield an essential oil with a very pleasant odour. This oil becomes viscous upon exposure to air.

Magnolia leaf oil contains about 3% of phenols, 4% of carbonyl compounds and some cineole and sesquiterpenes.

The scent of magnolia oil is related to that of orange flower and lily-of-the-valley oils. Natural magnolia oil is not available commercially and most fragrance formulations are synthetically compounded. The jasmine absolute constituent, 3-acetonyl-2-pentyl-1-cyclopentanone have a strong magnolia odour. The magnolia scent is fixed by orris concrete, Tolu balsam, tonka absolute and vanilla resinoid. Magnolia has been used as a single floral perfume by Chanel but it is more commonly used as a component in heavier floral perfumes like violet. Fragrances using magnolia in their formulation include Mystere and Cabriole.
[Perfumer & Flavourist (1992) Vol.17 No.2 pgs.27-9]

osmanthus oil (Osmanthus fragrans) Oleaceae
The osmanthus plant is native to China and Japan and is cultivated in three different varieties: golden flower (variety thunbergii); silver flower (variety latifolius) and reddish flower (variety aurantiacus). The composition of osmanthus oils varies slightly according to flower variety.

Composition of **golden flower osmanthus oil** - 1.5% nonanol, 6.5% linalool oxide, 2.9% linalool, 1.5% decanoic acid, 1.2% theaspirane, 4.5% p-methoxy b-phenylethyl alcohol, 2.2% a-ionone, 5.8% dihydro-b-ionol, 18.5% b-ionone, 1.6% dibutyl phthalate and 4.2% hexadecanoic acid.

Composition of **silver flower osmanthus oil** - 7.6% linalool oxide, 3.4% linalool, 1.6% p-methoxy b-phenylethyl alcohol, 6.5% a-ionone, 3.8% dihydro-b-ionol, 8.6% b-ionone, 3.4% g-decalactone, 4.2% dibutyl phthalate and 1.4% hexadecanoic acid.

Composition of **reddish flower osmanthus oil** - 1.3% nonanol, 2.6% linalool oxide, 1.8% linalool, 2.4% geraniol, 1.1% decanoic acid, 1.6% p-methoxy b-phenylethyl alcohol, 1.3% a-ionone, 3.7% dihydro-b-ionol, 9.2% b-ionone, 4.1% g-decalactone, 1% 4-oxo-b-ionol and 3.7% hexadecanoic acid. [Perfumer & Flavourist (1992) Vol.17 No.3 pgs.72-6]

hinoki oil (Chamaecyparis obtusa) Cupressaceae
The hinoki tree is a conifer found in Japan. Essential oils are distilled from the leaf and wood. Another species, C. taiwanensis grows in Taiwan. [Perfumer & Flavourist (1978) Vol.3 No.3 pgs.46]

Composition of **hinoki leaf oil** - 1% a-pinene, 1.6% sabinene, 2.8% b-pinene, 1% a-terpinene, 3% limonene, 1.8% g-terpinene, 1% terpinolene, 2% a-fenchol, 1.2% borneol, 1% a-terpineol, 7% bornyl acetate, 1.7% cis-caryophyllene, 4.7% b-cadrene, 1.5% a-elemene, 5.7% g-murolene, 9% a-terpinyl acetate, 3.8% a-murolene, 2.8% d-cadinene, 14.8% elemol, 8.3% g-eudesmol, 5.4% a-eudesmol, 6.5% b-eudesmol and 1.7% cadin-10(15)-4-ol.

Composition of **hinoki wood oil** - 1.7% g-murolene, 5.8% a-murolene, 10.8% d-cadinene, 12.5% g-cadinene, 1.5% b-caryophyllene alcohol, 10.6% t-cadinol, 18.5% t-murolol, 20.5% a-cadinol and 6.8% cadin-1(10)-3n-4-beta-ol. [Perfumer & Flavourist (1983) Vol.8 No.2 pgs.62-3]

Safety application for hinoki oil is tentatively assumed to be similar to that of hibawood oil. **The recommended limit of use is 12%**

kesom oil (Polygonum minus) Polygonaceae
Kesom is a strongly aromatic herb native to Malaysia that is popular with the local people as a flavouring spice. The leaves are cut into small pieces and subsequently dispersed into rice and noodle dishes. Sometimes the leaves are mixed with other local spices and used as stuffing for traditional foods. Steam distillation of the fresh leaves yields 0.3-0.4% of a colourless essential oil. The plant favours a wet soil and cool climate (15-24 degrees C.) for proper growth and a rich yield of essential oil. Specimens grown at the developed agricultural area of the Cameron Highlands at 1600m produced an essential oil richest in the two dominant aldehydes found in the oil, decanal and dodecanal. In the lowlands, kesom is grown in local villages for domestic use and for selling in the markets as a fresh herb spice.
Composition: 0.86% nonanal, 0.76% l-nonanol, 24.36% decanal, 2.5% l-decanol, 1.8% undecanal, 1.4% l-undecanol, 48.2% dodecanal, 0.18% b-caryophyllene, 2.44% l-dodecanol and 1.42% tetradecanal. [Perfumer & Flavourist (1987) Vol.12 No.5 pgs.27-30]
Safety application for kesom oil is undetermined at present.

Australia & New Guinea -

boronia absolute (Boronia megastigma) Rutaceae
Boronia is a woody shrub growing in the southwestern region of South Australia. The flowers are used to extract a highly priced absolute.
Composition: major constituents - dodecanol, dodecyl acetate, tetradecyl acetate and b-ionone, with a-pinene, camphene, b-pinene, myrcene, limonene, ocimene, linalool, a-ionone, dihydro-b-ionone and menthone. [Perfumer & Flavourist (1983) Vol.8 No.2 pgs.61]
Safety application for boronial absolute is undetermined at present.

massoia oil (Cryptocarya massoia) Lauraceae
The massoia tree is native to the island of New Guinea in South-East Asia, north of Australia. It is related to the cinnamon tree but the essential oil distilled from the bark has a warm aroma reminiscent of a mixture of coconut and peach. Massoia oil contains three unusual lactones.
Composition: 68.2% 6-pentyl-5,6-dihydro-2H-pyran-2-one, 14.6% 6-heptyl-5,6-dihydro-2H-pyran-2-one, 0.34% 6-nonyl-5,6-dihydro-2H-pyran-2-one and 8% benzyl benzoate.
[Perfumer & Flavourist (1984) Vol.9 No.2 pgs.24-6]
Safety application for massoia oil is undetermined at present.

South Africa -

layana oil (Artemisia afra) Compositae
Layana is a species of artemisia indigenous to South Africa growing throughout the Anatola and Drakensberg mountain regions. It is known locally as wildeals and the essential oil is steam distilled from the dried herbs collected from the wild by local tribesfolk, having odour similarities to armoise, wormwood and thuja leaf oils.

Composition: 1.15% camphene, 13% 1,8-cineole, 52.5% a-thujone, 13% b-thujone, 6.5% camphone, 2% artemisia ketone, 1.6% caryophyllene, 1.5% a-bergamotene and 1.4% aromadendrene. [Perfumer & Flavourist (1984) Vol.9 No.1 pgs.60]

The leaves and flowering tops yield 0.4% of an essential oil that is yellowish-brown to dark green in colour but as the azulene content increases the oil becomes blue-green. The local folk in Ciskei inhale layana oil for respiratory relief due to its medicinal note from the cineole and thujone. [Perfumer & Flavourist (1984) Vol.9 No.5 pgs.62]

The content of thujone and the ratio of the a- and b- isomers in layana oil is very similar to that of Moroccan armoise oil (A. herba-alba) and thuja leaf oil. Safety application for layana oil may be tentatively assumed to be comparable to both essential oils. **Recommended limit of use at 2%**

pteronia oil (Pteronia incana) Compositae

Pteronia is a perennial herb growing wild in the Ciskei province of South Africa. The essential oil possesses an odour reminiscent of a mixture of dwarf pine, Siberian fir leaf and cypress combined with a thujone note.

Composition: 32.5% b-pinene, 18.6% a-pinene, 11.3% p-cymene, 10.3% myrcene, 9% 1,8-cineole, 7.4% sabinene, 7.2% methyl eugenol, 7% limonene, 5.3% terpinen-4-ol, 3.2% b-caryophyllene, 3.1% ledene, 2.3% d-cadinene, 2.1% ar-curcumene, 1.3% trans-pinocarveol, 1.3% a-terpineol, 1.2% a-humulene, 1.2% bicyclo-germacrene and 1.1% a-murolene.
[Perfumer & Flavourist (1989) Vol.14 No.1 pgs.40-1]

Pteronia (pronounced teronia) is a small shrub having multi-branched stems and grey leaves growing prolifically in the Eastern Cape of South Africa. Steam distillation of the entire plant yields 0.3% of a pale yellow essential oil. [Perfumer & Flavourist (1984) Vol.9 No.5 pgs.63]
Safety application for pteronia oil is undetermined at present.

eriocephalus oil (Eriocephalus punctulatus) Compositae

Eriocephalus is a woody shrub or bush growing at elevations of 3000 metres on the slopes of the Lesotho mountains in South Africa. This plant has been used by the local inhabitants of Southern Lesotho to fumigate the hut of a person suffering from a cold or diarrhoea or when the person has died. It has also been used as a substitute for another local plant, buchu, by the native folk in the region where it is commonly found. The essential oil is steam distilled from the flowers, having a deep blue colour and possessing a powerful fruity fresh Roman chamomile-like odour. [Perfumer & Flavourist (1979) Vol.4 No.5 pgs.9 and (1983) Vol8 No.6 pgs.76]

Composition: 3.5-6% a-pinene, 1-2% b-pinene, 0.5-1% limonene, 3.5-8% p-cymene, 2-5% terpinen-4-ol and 0.5% a-terpineol, with 0.5% 2-methylbutan-1-ol, 0.1% 3-methylbutan-1-ol, 1% 2-methylbutyl butyrate, 14% 2-methylpropyl 2 methyl propionate, 22.6% 2-methylbutyl 2 methyl propionate, 3.6% 3-methylbutyl 2 methyl propionate, 1% 2-methylbutyl pentanoate, 1% 2-methylpropyl 3-methyl butyrate, 4.5% 2-methylbutyl 3-methyl butyrate.

The compounds responsible for the intense blue colour of the oil were found to be 0.32% 1,4-dimethyl azulene and 0.07% 1,4-dimethyl-7-ethyl azulene (chamazulene).

Known locally as sahalahala, the fleshy leaves of eriocephalus yield a deep yet bright blue essential oil with an azulene deriviative content up to 16%.
[Perfumer & Flavourist (1984) Vol.9 No.5 pgs.62-3]
Safety application for eriocephalus oil is undetermined at present.

buchu oil (Barosma betulina & crenulata) Rutaceae

Buchu is a native plant of South Africa, growing in the high altitude regions of the Western Cape Province. Buchu oil is obtained by steam distillation of the leaves. The main use of buchu oil is in compounding blackcurrant flavour, where it imparts unique and characteristic flavour and aroma qualities.

The essential oil contains sulphurated terpenoid ketones, including 8-mercapto-p. menthane-3-one, 8-acetylthio-p. menthane-3-one, which were important for the high flavour impact. The concentration of these compounds in the essential oil varies between the 2 species.
[Perfumer & Flavourist (1976) Vol.1 No.2 pgs.17]

Buchu is a small shrub having opposite leaves and white five petalled flowers. The leaves are picked and dried and formerly sent to Europe and the U.S. for distillation but is now distilled at source in South Africa to yield 1.0% of a dark brown essential oil possessing an exceptionally pungent phenolic-blackcurrant, semi-sweet, medicinal aroma which is mainly due to its content of diosphenol. [Perfumer & Flavourist (1984) Vol.9 N0.5 pgs.64]
Safety application for buchu oil is undetermined at presentl

East Africa -

muhuhu oil (Brachylaena hutchinsii) Compositae

Muhuhu is a moderately large tree growing in East Africa. The essential oil is obtained by steam distillation of the wood, possessing a sandalwood-vetivert-cedarwood aroma.

Composition: 1% a-ylangene, 2% a-copaene, 16.5% a-amophene, 3% a-murolene, 1% g-amorphene, 6.5% d-cadinene, 0.5% calamenene, 5% a-calcorene, 10% brachyl oxide, 4% ylangenal, 3.5% cubebol, 7.5% copaenal, 3% cadalene, 1.5% ylangenol, 7.5% copaenol, 4.5% cyclic ether and 5% sesquiterpene alcohol. [Perfumer & Flavourist (1980) Vol.5 No.2 pgs.36]
Safety application for muhuhu oil is undetermined at present.

South America -

amyris oil (Amyris balsamifera) Rutaceae
Amyris is a tree native to the Caribbean from which an essential oil is obtained possessing a weak, woody, sandalwood-like odour. The oil is produced mainly in Haiti for using as a fixative in soap fragrances. [Perfumer & Flavourist (1980) Vol.4 No.6 pgs.31]

Composition: 2.5% zingiberene, 1% b-dihydro-agarofuran, 4.7% b-sesquiphellendrene, 1.5% ar-curcumene, 2.5% selina-3,7(11)-diene, 9% elemol, 9.7% 10-epi-g-eudesmol, 6.6% g-eudesmol, 21.5% valerianol, 4.8% a-eudesmol, 10.7% 7-epi-a-eudesmol, 8% b-eudesmol, and 1% drimenol. [Perfumer & Flavourist (1990) Vol.15 No.2 pgs.78]

The United States NIOSH determined the oral toxicity of amyris oil to be 4.54g/kg. Amyris oil is included in the approved flavourings lists of both the United States FDA and the Council of Europe.

The RIFM only conducted safety tests for the acetylated form of amyris oil. Information on the safety of natural amyris oil is not yet available. Safety applications for amyris oil is tentatively assumed to be comparable to that for the acetylated form.
The recommended limit of use is at 10%.

ayou oil (Nectandra globosa) Lauraceae
The ayou tree is a tall tropical evergreen indigenous to French Guiana in South America. The essential oil is obtained by steam distillation from the wood chips, possessing a fresh, spicy, borneol aroma. When the phenols are removed, its smell has a more pleasant, intense, fresh, spicy wood character.

Composition: 2.8% a-pinene, 3.2% b-pinene, 2.8% borneol, 2.2% a-copaene, 2.5% trans-a-bergamotene & b-curcumene, 1.2% a-humulene & b-farnesene, 6.6% 1,11-oxidocalamenene & ar-curcumene, 2.9% sesqui-1,8-cineole & b-bisabolene, 1.8% g-cadinene, 2.1% cubebol & trans-calamenene, 5.8% d-cadinene & furopelargone A, 4% a-calacorene & trans-sesquisabinene hydrate, 6.5% (E)-nerolidol, 2% cis-sesquisabinene hydrate, 1.1% caryophyllene oxide, 3.4% guaiol, 1.1% 1,10-di-epi-cubenol, 2.7% 1-epi-cubenol, 1.3% selin-11-en-4-a-ol, 4.9% B-eudesmol & a-cadinol, 2.1% cubenol, 8.3% b-bisabolol, 3.7% benzyl benzoate and 1.6% benzyl salicylate. [Perfumer & Flavourist (1990) Vol.15 No.3 pgs.64]
Safety application for ayou oil is undetermined at present.

carqueja oil (Baccharis genistelloides) Compositae
Carqueja is a South American plant widely used as folk medicine in Brazil. A small quantity of essential oil is distilled from the whole plants and offered for sale each year.

Composition: 55-69.2% carquejyl acetate (o-mentha-1,7,5,8-trien-3-yl acetate), 6-7% carquejol (o-mentha-1,7,5,8-trien-3-ol) and 8.4% b-pinene, 6.4% a-pinene, 2.6% camphene, nopinene, ledol, myrcene, cis- and trans- ocimene. [Perfumer & Flavourist (1986) Vol.11 No.6 pgs.42]
Safety application for carqueja oil is undetermined at present.

vassoura oil (Baccharis dracunculifolia) Compositae
Vassoura is a South American shrub found uncultivated throughout central southern Brazil. The essential oil possesses a spicy, woody, peppery aroma.

Composition: 30% nerolidol, 11% b-pinene, 10.8% limonene, 5.5% farnesol and 3% a-pinene.
[Perfumer & Flavourist (1984) Vol.9 No.5 pgs.94-5]
Safety application for vassoura oil is undetermined at present.

cangerana oil (Cabralea cangerana) Meliaceae
The essential oil of cangerana is only produced in Brazil.
Composition: caryophyllene (major constituent), d-cadinene, g-murolene, b-elemene, d-elemene, a-copaene, daucalene, calacorene, guaiazulene, dihydroguaiazulene, safrole, isosafrole, caryophyllene-2,6-b-oxide, jujenol and juniper camphor. **No quantitative data was available**.
[Perfumer & Flavourist (1986) Vol.11 No.6 pgs.43]
Safety application for cangerana oil is undetermined at present.

cedro oil (Cedrela odorata) Meliaceae
Cedro is a Brazilian tree yielding timber for making cabinets and cigar boxes. The wood chips and sawdust are steam distilled to provide an essential oil possessing a characteristic dry-woody aroma with good tenacity.

Composition: 8% a-cubebene, 15.6% a-copaene, 3.2% b-cubenene, 6.8% b-curcumene, 11.7% d-cadinene, 1.3% cadina-1,4-diene, 3.4% calarene, 1.2% caryophyllene, 1.8% b-farnesene, 2.1% a-humulene, 2.6% germacrene D, 1% a-murolene, 8% (E)-nerolidol and 1.4% epi-cubenol.
[Perfumer & Flavourist (1987) vol.12 No.3 pgs.58-9]
Safety application for cedro oil is undetermined at present.

North America -

goldenrod oil (Solidago odora) Compositae
The goldenrod is a graceful plant blooming in late summer distributed from Newfoundland to West Virginia and Kentucky in North America. Steam distillation of the plant yields a yellowish essential oil smelling strongly of licorice. Goldenrod oil was formerly available together with mint oils, but production has now almost ceased.
[Perfumer & Flavourist (1979) Vol.3 No.6 pgs.33]
Safety application for goldenrod oil is undetermined at present.

heterotheca oil (Heterotheca latifolia) Compositae
Heterotheca is a composite weed with a camphoraceous smell, growing wild in North America. It has no known medicinal or economic value. Steam distillation of the air-dried plants produce an essential oil. The yield is quite low at 0.1% but the oil has an intense odour so small amounts are sufficient to produce the scent which is wild and spicy with a camphoraceous note also resembling armoise oil.

Composition: 3.7% a-pinene, 5.5% camphene, 6% b-pinene, 15% limonene, 1.8% g-terpinene, 1.4% trans-b-ocimene, 1% p-cymene, 2.2% bornyl acetate, 2% terpinen-4-ol, 1.5% b-caryophyllene, 21.4% borneol, 6.4% germacrene D and 1% d-cadinene.
[Perfumer & Flavourist (1986) Vol.11 No.5 pgs.67-8]
Safety application for heterotheca oil is undetermined at present.

erigeron oil (Erigeron canadensis) Compositae
Erigeron is a common weed in the midwestern United States, known locally as maretail. It is collected from the wild where it grows very profusely for distilling the essential oil in southern Michigan and northern Indiana. Erigeron oil had been used to a limited extent in pharmaceutical preparations but is not now readily available.
[Perfumer & Flavourist (1979) Vol.3 No.6 pgs.33]
Safety application for erigeron oil is undetermined at present.

monarda oil (Monarda fistulosa) Labiatae
Monarda is a perennial and somewhat hardy herb native to North America. Steam distillation of the fresh plant produces an essential oil with a yield ranging from 0.5 - 0.8% according to the vigour and condition of the plants. Monarda oil is very rich in geraniol at over 90%. The leaves and flower heads yield the highest amount of essential oil but the geraniol content of the oil is lower than that from the petals and stems. Overall the geraniol content is very stable despite varying growing conditions. [Perfumer & Flavourist (1982) Vol.7 No.3 pgs.32-4]
Safety application for monarda oil is undetermined at present.

tuberose absolute (Polianthus tuberosa) Agavaceae
The tuberose is a plant native to Mexico. Solvent of the tuberose flower produces an absolute that is among the most desirable and expensive perfumery raw materials. Two and a half million fully bloomed flowers weighing about 2 tons will produce about 1 kilo of concrete which is then used to extract a very small amount of the absolute. Tuberose absolute is yellowish brown in colour possessing an overpowering, narcotically potent sweet floral scent.
Composition: major components include methyl benzoate, methyl anthranilate, geraniol, nerol and farnesol. [Perfumer & Flavourist (1984) Vol.9 No.5 pgs.62]

Chapter 9

Summary and Quick Reference Table

The general guide for calculating the concentration of essential oils to be blended with fixed oils for use in aromatherapy treatments is to decrease the dosage with an increase in the area of body surface that the essential oils are applied to. For application to the whole body in a massage, the usual concentration is between 2 - 5%. For smaller areas of the body, higher concentrations may be used. Generally 10% may be used for the area of the chest or abdomen. For smaller areas such as the hands and feet, up to 50% may be used. For applying topically to a spot, some essential oils may be used pure at 100% without diluting. At whatever concentration that is used, the total quantity or essential oils should be kept at approximately 0.5 - 1.5ml (10 - 30 drops).

These values are calculated for adults. When treating children, the dosages have to be reduced accordingly. The general guide is to use half a drop of essential oil for each kg of the child's weight. Otherwise calculate as a fraction of the adult dosage. 12 - 16 years old: one half to two-thirds (10 - 15 drops)
> 7 - 12 years old: one quarter to one third (5 - 8 drops)
> 3 - 7 years old: one sixth (3 drops)
> 1 - 3 years old: one twentieth (1 drop)
> under 1 year old: do not use.

The usual frequency of aromatherapy treatments involving a full body massage with the essential oil blends is between once a week to once a month. Some individuals may for a period have up to three massage treatments or aromatic baths using essential oils, a week. The tolerance of using essential oils also very much depends on the state of the individual at the time. Individuals who are new to aromatherapy treatments need to allow their bodies to get accustomed to the essential oils.

The following table is a summary of the information presented in Chapters 7 and 8 for a quick reference to the recommended limit of use without the accompanying texts. The values indicated here are not absolute. Many essential oils can be used safely above the level recommended here, but the recommended levels are those that are known from controlled studies to be generally safe. They are intended to provide a general guide. Individuals still have to use their own judgement to evaluate the actual situation when using the essential oils.

Reference Table - for application on the skin

Recommended limit of use of the essential oils:

20%

bergamot oil, rectified (Citrus bergamia) Rutaceae
camphor oil, white (Cinnamomum camphora) Lauraceae
fir cone oil, silver (Abies alba) Pinaceae
fir needle oil, silver (Abies alba) Pinaceae

15%

lavender oil (Lavandula officinalis) Labiatae
lime oil, distilled (Citrus aurantifolia) Rutaceae

10%

hibawood oil (Thujopsis dolabrata) Cupressaceae
hinoki oil (Chamaecyparis obtusa) Cupressaceae - *tentative*
pine oil, Scots (Pinus sylvestris) Pinaceae
bois de rose oil (Aniba rosaedora) Lauraceae
sandalwood oil (Santalum album) Santalaceae
agarwood oil (Aquilaria agallocha) Thymelaceae - *tentative*
patchouli oil (Pogostemon cablin) Labiatae
spikenard oil (Nardostachys jatamansi) Valerianaceae - *tentative*
ylang-ylang oil (Cananga odorata) Annonaceae
cananga oil (Cananga odorata) Annonaceae
rosemary oil (Rosmarinus officinalis) Labiatae
fir needle oil, Canadian (Abies balsamea) Pinaceae
lemon oil, distilled (Citrus limon) Rutaceae
petitgrain oil, lemon (Citrus limon) Rutaceae
amyris oil (Amyris balsamifera) Rutaceae - *tentative*
(Eucalyptus globulus) oil. Myrtaceae
(Eucalyptus citriodora) oil. Myrtaceae

geranium oil, Algerian (Pelargonium graveolens) Geraniaceae
geranium oil, Bourbon (Pelargonium graveolens) Geraniaceae
geranium oil, Moroccan (Pelargonium graveolens) Geraniaceae

grapefruit oil, expressed (Citrus paradisi) Rutaceae - **mild phototoxic potential**
sweet orange oil, expressed (Citrus sinensis) Rutaceae - **mild phototoxic potential**
tangerine oil, expressed (Citrus reticulata) Rutaceae
mandarin oil, expressed (Citrus nobilis) Rutaceae

ho leaf oil (Cinnamomum camphora) Lauraceae
cinnamon leaf oil (Cinnamomum zeylanicum) Lauraceae
tejpat oil (Cinnamomum tamala) Lauraceae - *tentative*
bay oil (Pimenta racemosa) Myrtaceae

8%

lemonmint oil (Mentha citrata) Labiatae
cornmint oil (Mentha arvensis) Labiatae
sage oil, Spanish (Salvia lavendulaefolia) Labiatae
sage oil, clary French (Salvia sclarea) Labiatae
sage oil, clary Russian (Salvia sclarea) Labiatae
sage, Dalmatian (Salvia officinalis) Labiatae
spike lavender oil (Lavandula latifolia) Labiatae
thyme oil, garden red (Thymus vulgaris) Labiatae
thyme oil, wild (Thymus serpyllum) Labiatae - *tentative*
Spanish oregano oil (Thymus capitatus) Labiatae - *tentative*
ajowan oil (Trachyspermum ammi) Umbelliferae - *tentative*
labdanum oil (Cistus ladaniferus) Cistaceae
palmarosa oil (Cymbopogon martini) Graminae
vetivert oil (Vetiveria zizanoides) Graminae

bitter orange oil, expressed (Citrus aurantium) Rutaceae - **phototoxic potential**
lemon oil, expressed (Citrus limon) Rutaceae - **weak phototoxic potential**
tangelo oil, expressed (Citrus reticulata x paradisi) Rutaceae
petitgrain oil, Bigarade (Citrus aurantium) Rutaceae
petitgrain oil, Paraguay (Citrus aurantium) Rutaceae
linaloe wood oil (Bursera delpechiana) Burseraceae
guaiac wood oil (Bulnesia sarmienti) Zygophyllaceae
copaiba oil (Copaifera reticulata) Leguminosae
juniper berry oil (Juniperus communis) Cupressaceae

cubeb oil (Piper cubeba) Piperaceae
litsea oil (Litsea cubeba) Lauraceae - **slight sensitisation potential**
gurjun oil (Dipterocarpus turbinatus) Dipterocarpaceae
cedarwood oil, Atlas (Cedrus atlantica) Pinaceae

mace oil (Myristica fragrans) Myristicaceae
Peru balsam oil (Myroxylon pereirae) Leguminosae
myrrh oil (Commiphora myrrha) Burseraceae
olibanum oil (Boswellia carterii) Burseraceae - *tentative*

4%

Spanish marjoram oil (Thymus mastichiana) Labiatae
lavandin oil (Lavandula hybrida) Labiatae
cypress oil (Cupressus sempervirens) Cupressaceae
cabreuva oil (Murocarpus frondosus) Leguminosae
chamomile oil, German (Matricaria chamomilla) Compositae
chamomile oil, Roman (Anthemis nobilis) Compositae
yarrow oil (Achillea millefolium) Compositae - *tentative*
davana oil (Artemisia pallens) Compositae
immortelle oil (Helichrysum angustifolium) Compositae

lemongrass oil, E. Indian (Cymbopogon citratus) Graminae
lemongrass oil, W. Indian (Cymbopogon citratus) Graminae
cardamon oil (Elettaria cardamomum) Zingiberaceae
galangal oil (Alpinia galanga) Zingiberaceae - *tentative*
turmeric oil (Curcuma longa) Zingiberaceae
ginger oil (Zingiber officinale) Zingiberaceae- **mild phototoxic & irritation potential**
pepper oil (Piper nigrum) Piperaceae - **mild phototoxic potential**
lime oil, expressed (Citrus aurantifolia) Rutaceae - **strong phototoxic potential**
carrot seed oil (Daucus carota) Umbelliferae
celery seed oil (Apium graveolens) Umbelliferae
fennel seed oil, bitter (Foeniculum vulgare) Umbelliferae
fennel seed oil, sweet (Foeniculum vulgare) Umbelliferae
dill seed oil, Indian (Anethum sowa) Umbelliferae
dill herb oil (Anethum graveolens) Umbelliferae
galbanum oil (Ferula galbaniflua) Umbelliferae
spearmint oil (Mentha spicata) Labiatae
peppermint oil (Mentha piperita) Labiatae - *tentative*
neroli/orange flower oil (Citrus aurantium) Rutaceae

myrtle oil (Myrtus communis) Myrtaceae
Peruvian mastic oil (Schinus molle) Anacardiaceae
cascarilla oil (Croton elutheria) Euphorbiaceae
snakeroot oil (Asarum canadensis) Aristolochiaceae

coriander oil (Coriandrum sativum) Umbelliferae
cajeput oil (Melaleuca leucodendron) Myrtaceae
flouve oil (Anthoxanthum odoratum) Graminae

elemi oil (Canarium commune) Burseraceae
clove bud oil (Eugenia caryophyllata) Myrtaceae
clove stem oil (Eugenia caryophyllata) Myrtaceae
star anise oil (Illicium verum) Illiciaceae

marjoram oil (Origanum marjorana) Labiatae
tarragon oil (Artemisia dracunculus) Compositae
birch oil, sweet (Betula lenta) Betulaceae

chervil oil (Anthriscus cerefolium) Umbelliferae - *tentative*
pine oil, yarmour (Pinus palustris) Pinaceae

basil oil (Ocimum basilicum) Labiatae
hyssop oil (Hyssopus officinalis) Labiatae
tansy oil (Tanacetum vulgare) Compositae

caraway oil (Carum carvi) Umbelliferae - **moderate dermal toxicity**
pimento leaf oil (Pimenta officinalis) Myrtaceae - **moderate dermal toxicity**
pimento berry oil (Pimenta officinalis) Myrtaceae - **moderate dermal toxicity**

2%

birch tar oil (Betula pendula) Betulaceae
cade tar oil (Juniperus oxycedrus) Cupressaceae

rose oil, Bulgarian (Rosa damascena) Rosaceae
rose oil, Turkish (Rosa damascena) Rosaceae
rose oil, Moroccan (Rosa centifolia) Rosaceae

bergamot oil, expressed (Citrus bergamia) Rutaceae - **severe phototoxic potential**

parsley seed oil (Petroselinum sativum) Umbelliferae
parsley herb oil (Petroselinum sativum) Umbelliferae
lovage oil (Levisticum officinale) Umbelliferae

laurel leaf oil (Laurus nobilis) Lauraceae
nutmeg oil (Myristica fragrans) Myristicaceae

anise oil (Pimpinella anisum) Umbelliferae
wormwood oil (Artemisia absinthum) Compositae
santolina oil (Santolina chamaecyparissus) Compositae - *tentative*

thuja leaf oil (Thuja occidentalis) Cupressaceae - **high oral toxicity**
armoise oil (Artemisia vulgaris) Compositae - **high oral toxicity**
layana oil (Artemisia afra) Compositae - *tentative*
pennyroyal oil (Mentha pulegium) Labiatae - **high oral toxicity**

cumin oil (Cuminum cyminum) Umbelliferae - **strong phototoxic potential**
clove leaf oil (Eugenia caryophyllata) Myrtaceae - **moderate dermal toxicity**

1%

ambrette seed oil (Hibiscus ablemoschus) Malvaceae
juniper oil, Phoenician (Juniperus phoenicia) Cupressaceae
fir needle oil, Siberian (Abies sibirica) Pinaceae
angelica seed oil (Angelica archangelica) Umbelliferae
spruce oil (Picea mariana) Pinaceae

tea tree oil (Melaleuca alternifolia) Myrtaceae

T. cedarwood oil (Juniperus mexicana) Cupressaceae - **irritation & sensitisation**
V. cedarwood oil (Juniperus virginiana) Cupressaceae - **irritation & phototoxic**
pine oil, pumilo (Pinus pumio) Pinaceae - **irritation potential**
citronella oil (Cymbopogon nardus) Graminae - **irritation potential**

angelica root oil (Angelica archangelica) Umbelliferae - **severe phototoxic potential**

cassia oil (Cinnamomum aromaticum) Lauraceae - **moderate sensitisation potential**
cinnamon bark oil (Cinnamomum zeylanicum) Lauraceae - **sensitisation potential**

0.5%

perilla oil (Perilla frutescens) labiatae - **irritation potential**
rue oil (Ruta graveolens) Rutaceae - **severe phototoxic potential**
oregano oil (Origanum vulgare) Labiatae - **high dermal toxicity**
savory oil (Satureja hortensis) Labiatae - **high dermal toxicity**

0.25%

tagetes oil (Tagetes minuta) Compositae - **irritation and sensitisation potential**
verbena oil (Lippia citriodora) Verbenaceae - **sensitisation and phototoxic potential**

0.1%

costus root oil (Sassurea lappa) Compositae - **severe sensitisation potential**
elecampane root oil (Inula helenium) Compositae - **severe sensitisation potential**

best not be used

camphor oil, yellow (Cinnamomum camphora) Lauraceae - **carcinogenic potential**
camphor oil, brown (Cinnamomum camphora) Lauraceae - **carcinogenic potential**
sassafras oil (Sassafras albidum) Lauraceae - **carcinogenic potential**
Brazilian sassafras oil (Ocotea cymbarum) Lauraceae - **carcinogenic potential**

calamus oil (Acorus calamus) Araceae - **carcinogenic potential**

mustard oil (Brassica nigra) Cruciferae - **very strong irritation potential**
horseradish oil (Amoracia rusticana) Cruciferae - **very strong irritation potential**

bitter almond oil (Prunus amygadalus) Rosaceae [FFPA] - **oral and dermal toxicity**
bitter almond oil (Prunus amygadalus) Rosaceae - **high oral and dermal toxicity**

wintergreen oil (Gaultheria procumbens) Ericaceae - **high oral & dermal toxicity**
chenopodium oil (Chenopodium ambrosioides) Chenopodiaceae **very high toxicity**
boldo leaf oil (Peumus boldus) Monimiaceae - **very high oral and dermal toxicity**
savin oil (Juniperus sabina) Cupressaceae - **very high oral & dermal toxicity**

of yet undetermined safety

melissa oil (Melissa officinalis) Labiatae
monarda oil (Monarda fistulosa) Labiatae
goldenrod oil (Solidago odora) Compositae
muhuhu oil (Brachylaena hutchinsii) Compositae
heterotheca oil (Heterotheca latifolia) Compositae
balsamite oil (Chrysanthemum balsamite) Compositae
eriocephalus oil (Eriocephalus punctulatus) Compositae
vassoura oil (Baccharis dracunculifolia) Compositae
carqueja oil (Baccharis genistelloides) Compositae
actractylis oil (Actractylodes lancea) Compositae
erigeron oil (Erigeron canadensis) Compositae
pteronia oil (Pteronia incana) Compositae
blumea oil (Blumea mollis) Compositae
asafoetida oil (Ferula asafoetida) Umbelliferae
parsnip root oil (Pastinaca sativa) Umbelliferae
ammoniac gum oil (Dorema ammoniacum) Umbelliferae
zdravetz oil (Geranium macrorrhizum) Geraniaceae
valerian oil (Valerian officinalis) Valerianaceae
licorice oil (Glycyrrihza glabra) Leguminosae
cassie oil (Acacia farnesiana) Leguminosae
skimmia oil (Skimmia laureola) Rutaceae
buchu oil (Barosma betulina) Rutaceae
ayou oil (Nectandra globosa) Lauraceae
massoia oil (Cryptocarya massoia) Lauraceae
gardenia oil (Gardenia jasminoides) Rubiaceae
lily-of-the-valley oil (convallaria majalis) Liliaceae
carnation oil (Dianthus caryophyllus) Caryophyllaceae
magnolia oil (Magnolia grandiflora) Magnoliaceae
osmanthus oil (Osmanthus fragrans) Oleaceae
lilac oil (Syringa vulgaris) Oleaceae
cedro oil (Cedrela odorata) Meliaceae
cangerana oil (Cabralea cangerana) Meliaceae
blackcurrant bud oil (Ribes nigrum) Rosaceae
vateria oil (Vateria indica) Dipterocarpaceae
mignonette oil (Reseda odorata) Resedaceae
kesom oil (Polygonum minus) Polygonaceae
abutilon oil (Abutilon indicum) Malvaceae

Chapter 10

General Advice on the Use of Essential Oils in Aromatherapy

Aromatic essences commonly sold in shops as 'essential oils' for use in aromatherapy are natural plant products. They occur naturally in plants at very low concentrations. Most vary between 0.1 - 1.0% while some occur at concentrations as low as 0.01%.

When they are extracted from the plants and bottled as pure essential oils, the concentration is 100%. At this concentration, their potency is 100 - 1000 times stronger than in their naturally occurring state. They are available in the pure form for purchase by the public and when used for self-help or for domestic application, should be adequately diluted for safety.

When properly used, essential oils are beneficial in helping with various health problems. However, like all biologically active substances, they are not risk free, and misuse may cause severe adverse reactions.

A generally safe concentration is 2% diluted in fixed oils (such as olive or almond oils), with an upper limit of 5% when used for massage on the whole body. It is important to understand that unnecessary increase in concentration does not correspond to an increase in effectiveness. If used in the bath, a maximum of 8 drops in a full bathtub of water is usually adequate for the desired effect with minimal risk of adverse reactions. The addition of an emulsifier like liquid soap or bath salts will also reduce irritation to the eyes.

The reaction of different individuals to the essential oils when applied to the body varies enormously, and some hypersensitive individuals will be allergic to even miniscule amounts. This does not make the essential oils dangerous to everyone. If possible sensitivity is uncertain, start with a very low concentration and gradually increase to the recommended 2%.

It is generally not recommended to ingest the essential oils orally because of the complications and risks involved in doing so by the inexperienced.

However anyone wishing to do so should understand that all essential oils are irritants to the mucous membranes and are practically insoluble in water. It is therefore hazardous to attempt to drink essential oils mixed in water-based beverages (or to swallow them in sugar lumps as may be suggested in some literature). Honey is also useless as an excipient. To do so will cause the essential oils to burn the mucous lining of the gastro-intestinal tract. The only suitable vehicles for ingesting essential oils are alcohol (ethanol) and glycerol.

The standard pharmacopoeial recommendation for oral ingestion is either as a spirit (10% essential oil in 90% ethanol) or as a concentrated water (2% essential oil in 60% ethanol and 38% water). Both preparations are intended to be further diluted before ingesting in doses from 0.3 - 1.2ml. Excessive doses of essential oils will cause nausea, vomiting and diarrhoea. Severe poisoning will lead to convulsions or respiratory failure.

Like all medicines, the pure essential oils should be kept out of reach of children or those liable to harm themselves through ignorance or carelessness.

When in doubt about what to do with essential oils, it is always prudent to consult professionals trained in their use. Unfortunately, the standard of aromatherapy training in the United Kingdom varies widely and not all aromatherapists will necessarily offer the same advice. Individuals who wish to use essential oils still have to be responsible for themselves and if sensible in their actions, will benefit greatly.

Aromatic plants are generally of low toxicity when considered in the context of the whole plant kingdom.

The most poisonous plant in the world (of the 250,000 known species of flowering plants) is recognised to be the Himalayan monkshood (Aconitum ferox) Ranunculaceae, found in northern India that produces the celebrated bikh poison. The toxic alkaloid, nepaline occurs at only 0.2%. This plant is so poisonous that it can kill just by being in close proximity. At a distance where it can be smelt, its poison will enter the body through inhalation. On contact, by touching the plant with any exposed part of the body, its poison readily enters the body through the skin. Initial symptoms start with tingling of the tongue, mouth, stomach and skin, followed by numbness and anaesthesia and muscular weakness. The poison affects both the heart and lungs and the central nervous system. Respiration is depressed and the heart is affected directly and through the vagus nerve, increasing in excitability and disturbance in its coordination and eventually stopping. The toxic effect is very rapid occurring within an hour, and death is almost instantaneous resulting from circulatory and respiratory failure. There is no specific antidote for monkshood poisoning. [Grieve 1931, Schauenberg & Paris 1974, Cooper & Johnson 1984] It has formerly been used in medicine but is an extremely dangerous therapeutic agent due to the closeness of its therapeutic and toxic doses and should only be used in homeopathic dilutions. [Martindale's Extra-Pharmacopoeia 28th ed. 1982]

Chapter 11

Safety of Aromatherapy in Pregnancy

Any drug treatment is always a balance of benefits and risks for the individual treated. However, during pregnancy, mothers become more vulnerable to certain drugs. Additionally the baby is also at risk from drug treatment during this period as certain drugs can cross over the placenta from the mother to the baby affecting development and growth. The effect of any substance on a pregnant woman also depends on her mental and physical condition. A mother will be more prone to the adverse effects of drugs if she has poor nutrition, is excessively overweight, is an alcoholic, a drug addict, a smoker or suffers from a chronic disease such as diabetes or high blood pressure.

Alcohol is hazardous to a pregnant woman and her baby. Regular daily use during the first 3 months will damage the baby; during the last 6 months, it will retard the baby's growth and during the last 3 months it may cause addiction in the baby so that the newborn baby of an alcoholic mother may develop withdrawal symptoms.

There are many problems in the study of the damaging effects of drug treatment in pregnancy. It is therefore very difficult to predict which drugs may cause damage to an unborn child. The molecular structure of drugs cannot provide any clues to their potential dangers as drugs with similar chemical structures may or may not produce congenital abnormalities. There is no direct relationship between the chemical structure of a drug and its effects on the pregnant woman or its specific damaging effects on the unborn baby. Also, observations of the damaging effects of drugs on pregnant animals also do not always suggest similar effects on pregnant women.

Because of these many difficulties, there is no convincing evidence from adequate and well controlled studies of the safety of many drugs used in medicine for treating pregnant women. Despite all these problems and warnings, pharmaceutical drugs appear to account for only about 1-5% of the 20,000 babies born with an abnormality each year in the U.K. [Parish 1991]

A normal term of pregnancy is usually about 9 months. This can be divided into 3 periods of 3 months each referred to as the first, second and third trimesters. The most critical period for the baby during pregnancy is the first trimester.

During this period, the baby is more sensitive to harmful effects in its environment than at any other time in its life. It is best to avoid using any drugs during this critical period, unless prescribed under medical supervision.

There is no evidence that any fragrance material is mutagenic (causing deformity) or teratogenic (causing monstrous growths) to the developing baby. The RIFM is confident enough about this situation to consider tests for these hazards as unnecessary. However minor problems may occur in vulnerable pregnant women when using certain essential oils.

Aromatherapy treatments during pregnancy are best performed by aromatherapists who also have experience in midwifery or in treating pregnant women. Individual aromatherapists may have safely used various essential oils in a specific way. However for the inexperienced, the general guideline to minimise the risks, is tentatively to avoid using all essential oils except the few that have been generally shown to be safe. Use at 0.5 - 1% (half the normal dosage).

The most suitable essential oils to use during pregnancy are the citrus essential oils, expressed or distilled - **bergamot oil, lime oil, lemon oil, bitter orange oil, petitgrain oil, neroli oil, sweet orange oil, grapefruit oil, tangerine oil and mandarin oil**. The last 2 are the best general purpose essential oils for pregnancy. (Observe phototoxic precautions for those oils with this hazard).

Other suitable essential oils to use during pregnancy are the gentler essential oils such as **geranium oil, sandalwood oil, chamomile oils (both), lavender oil, olibanum oil and rose oil.** All the above essential oils have been shown in practice to be generally safe for using throughout the entire term of pregnancy.

All these indicated essential oils are suitable for gentle massage on pregnant women. Additionally other essential oils may be used for inhalation including - **rosemary oil, spearmint oil, cajeput oil, eucalyptus oil and white camphor oil.**

Any essential oil that is known to stimulate menstruation should not be used for massage, particularly during the first trimester of pregnancy. Many other essential oils with intermediate potency may be included in treatments during pregnancy by those trained in their use. Certainly none of the essential oils indicated as hazardous in general, should be used during pregnancy.

As more information becomes available, confirming the safety of other essential oils for use in pregnancy, they can be added to the recommended list.

Chapter 12

Fragrance Materials Safety Listing

This is a complete listing of all the 250 fragrance materials described in this book, except for the 2 spurious essential oils and the 4 modified fragrance materials on page 109, which have been omitted. This listing is arranged alphabetically and also serves as an index. Page numbers where all the entries are found in the main section of the book in Chapters 7 & 8 are included. It is intended for the reader to simply check the recommended safe levels of use (when available) for any of the fragrance materials. If the reader wishes to look up more information, then the page numbers included will indicate where the information can be found.

Ten different concentrations are used for the recommended level of use for the essential oils -

20%   15%   10%   8%   4%   2%   1%   0.5%   0.25%   0.1%

The recommended values have been streamlined and follows the division in Chapter 9 for simplicity. The RIFM tested only one item (lavender oil) at 16% and another item (distilled lime oil) at 15%. 52 fragrance materials were tested at 4% while only 8 were tested at 5% and 5 were tested at 6%. They are now all listed under the next closest value according to the ten concentrations above.

The recommended levels for all the absolutes are listed at 3% or below; and for the balsams at 5% or below. These are the only exceptions to the divisions above

When the values are indicated as tentative, they were not determined by the RIFM but based on other information. These values may be revised when safety monographs are published for the respective fragrance materials in future. When the recommendation is indicated as uncertain, then the safe level of use cannot yet be determined from the available information.

The few floral essential oils included in this listing will probably not be obtained in sufficient quantities to become commercially available for a long time, if at all. No safety information is available for them and they are indicated as not important for this reason.

Plant Fragrance Materials	Recommended limit for safe use (%)
001 abutilon oil (Abutilon indicum) Malvaceae (pg125)	uncertain
002 actractylis oil (Actractylodes lancea) Compositae (pg126)	uncertain
003 agarwood oil (Aquillaria agallocha) Thymelaceae (pg123)	(tentative) 8.0
004 ajowan oil (Trachyspermum ammi) Umbelliferae (pg126)	(tentative) 8.0
005 almond oil, bitter (Prunus amygdalus) Rosaceae (pg96)	**do not use**
006 almond oil, bitter (Prunus amygdalus) Rosaceae [FFPA] (pg96)	**do not use**
007 ambrette seed oil (Hibiscus ablemoschus) Malvaceae (pg72)	1.0
008 ammoniac gum oil (Dorema ammoniacum) Umbelliferae (pg125)	uncertain
009 amyris oil (Amyris balsamifera) Rutaceae (pg131)	(tentative) 10.0
010 angelica root oil (Angelica archangelica) Umbelliferae (pg88)	1.0
011 angelica seed oil (Angelica archangelica) Umbelliferae (pg73)	1.0
012 anise oil (Pimpinella anisum) Umbelliferae (pg80)	2.0
013 armoise oil (Artemisia vulgaris) Compositae (pg84)	10.0
014 asafoetida oil (Ferula asafoetida) Umbelliferae (pg125)	uncertain

015 ayou oil (Nectandra globosa) Lauraceae (pg131)	uncertain
016 balsamite oil (Chrysanthemum balsamita) Compositae (pg114)	uncertain
017 basil oil, sweet (Ocimum basilicum) Labiatae (pg82)	4.0
018 bay oil (Pimenta racemosa) Myrtaceae (pg81)	10.0
019 benzoin resinoid (Styrax benzoin) Styracaceae (pg104)	3.0
020 bergamot oil, expressed (Citrus bergamia) Rutaceae (pg75)	2.0
021 bergamot oil, rectified (Citrus bergamia) Rutaceae (pg61)	20.0
022 birch tar oil (Betula pendula) Betulaceae (pg72)	2.0
023 sweet birch oil (Betula lenta) Betulaceae (pg81)	4.0
024 blackcurrant bud oil (Riges nigrum) Rosaceae (pg122)	uncertain
025 blumea oil (Blumea mollis) Compositae (pg126)	uncertain
026 bois de rose oil (Aniba rosaeodora) Lauraceae (pg76)	10.0
027 boldo leaf oil (Peumus boldus) Monimiaceae (pg97)	**do not use**
028 boronia oil (Boronia megastigma) Rutaceae (pg128)	uncertain
029 Brazilian sassafras oil (Ocotea cymbarum) Lauraceae (pg93)	**do not use**
030 buchu oil (Barosma betulina) Rutaceae (pg130)	uncertain

031 cabreuva oil (Murocarpus frondosus) Leguminosae (pg71)	4.0
032 cade tar oil (Juniperus oxycedrus) Cupressaceae (pg72)	2.0
033 cajeput oil (Melaleuca leucodendron) Myrtaceae (pg76)	4.0
034 calamus oil (Acorus calamus) Araceae (pg95)	**do not use**
035 camphor oil, white (Cinnamomum camphora) Lauraceae (pg61)	20.0
036 camphor oil, yellow (Cinnamomum camphora) Lauraceae (pg93)	**do not use**
037 camphor oil, brown (Cinnamomum camphora) Lauraceae (pg93)	**do not use**
038 cangerana oil (Cabralea cangerana) Meliaceae (pg132)	uncertain
039 cananga oil (Cananga odorata) Annonaceae (pg63)	10.0
040 caraway oil (Carum carvi) Umbelliferae (pg91)	4.0
041 cardamom oil (Elettaria cardamomum) Zingiberaceae (pg69)	4.0
042 carqueja oil (Baccharis genistelloides) Compositae (pg131)	uncertain
043 carnation oil (Dianthus caryophyllus) Caryophyllaceae (pg121)	not important
044 carrot seed oil (Daucus carota) Umbelliferae (pg69)	4.0
045 cascarilla oil (Croton eluteria) Euphorbiaceae (pg68)	4.0

046 cassia oil (Cinnamomum cassia) Lauraceae (pg90)	1.0
047 cassie oil (Acacia farnesiana) Leguminosae (pg121)	uncertain
048 cedarwood oil, Atlas (Cedrus atlantica) Pinaceae (pg66)	8.0
049 cedro oil (Cedrela odorata) Meliaceae (pg132)	uncertain
050 celery seed oil (Apium graveolens) Umbelliferae (pg69)	4.0
051 chamomile oil, German (Matricaria chamomilla) Compositae (pg67)	4.0
052 chamomile oil, Roman (Anthemis nobilis) Compositae (pg67)	4.0
053 chenopodium oil (Chenopodium ambrosioides) Chenopodiaceae (pg97)	**do not use**
054 chervil oil (Anthriscus cerefolium) Umbelliferae (pg115)	(tentative) 4.0
055 cinnamon bark oil (Cinnamomum zeylanicum) Lauraceae (pg90)	1.0
056 cinnamon leaf oil (Cinnamomum zeylanicum) Lauraceae (pg79)	10.0
057 citronella oil (Cymbopogon nardus) Graminae (pg87)	1.0
058 clove bud oil (Eugenia caryophyllata) Myrtaceae (pg79)	4.0
059 clove leaf oil (Eugenia caryophyllata) Myrtaceae (pg91)	2.0
060 clove stem oil (Eugenia caryophyllata) Myrtaceae (pg79)	4.0
061 copaiba balsam (Copaifera reticulata) Leguminosae (pg107)	5.0
062 copaiba oil (Copaifera reticulata) Leguminosae (pg65)	8.0
063 coriander oil (Coriandrum sativum) Umbelliferae (pg76)	4.0

064 cornmint oil (Mentha arvensis) Labiatae (pg82)	8.0
065 costus root absolute (Saussurea lappa) Compositae (pg105)	**do not use**
066 costus root oil (Saussurea lappa) Compositae (pg90)	0.1
067 cubeb oil (Piper cubeba) Piperaceae (pg66)	8.0
068 cumin oil (Cuminum cyminum) Umbelliferae (pg)	2.0
069 cypress oil (Cupressus sempervirens) Cupressaceae (pg71)	4.0
070 davana oil (Artemisia pallens) Compositae (pg67)	4.0
071 deertongue absolute (Liatris odoratissima) Compositae (pg100)	3.0
072 deertongue incolore (Liatris odoratissima) Compositae (pg103)	3.0
073 dill herb oil (Anethum graveolens) Umbelliferae (pg76)	4.0
074 dill seed oil, Indian (Anethum sowa) Umbelliferae (pg70)	4.0
075 Douglas fir balsam (Pseudotsuga taxifolia) Pinaceae (pg107)	5.0
076 eau de brouts absolute (Citrus aurantium) Rutaceae (pg99)	3.0
077 elecampane oil (Inula helenium) Compositae (pg90)	0.1
078 elemi oil (Canarium commune) Burseraceae (pg78)	4.0
079 erigeron oil (Erigeron canadensis) Compositae (pg133)	uncertain

080 eriocephalus oil (Eriocephalus punctulatus) Compositae (pg129)   uncertain

081 (Eucalyptus globulus) oil. Myrtaceae (pg64)   10.0
082 (Eucalyptus citriodora) oil. Myrtaceae (pg74)   10.0

083 fennel seed oil, bitter (Foeniculum vulgare) Umbelliferae (pg70)   4.0
084 fennel seed oil, sweet (Foeniculum vulgare) Umbelliferae (pg77)   4.0

085 fenugreek absolute (Trigonella foenum-graecum) Leguminosae (pg101) 2.0

086 fig leaf absolute (Ficus carica) Moraceae (pg105)   **do not use**

087 fir cone oil, silver (Abies alba) Pinaceae (pg62)   20.0
088 fir needle oil, silver (Abies alba) Pinaceae (pg62)   20.0
089 fir balsam, Canadian (Abies balsamea) Pinaceae (pg107)   2.0
090 fir needle oil, Canadian (Abies balsamea) Pinaceae (pg63)   10.0
091 fir needle oil, Siberian (Abies sibirica) Pinaceae (pg73)   1.0

092 flouve oil (Anthoxanthum odoratum) Graminae (pg77)   4.0
093 foin absolute (Anthoxanthum odoratum) Graminae (pg99)   3.0

094 galangal oil (Alpinia galanga) Zingiberaceae (pg123)   (tentative) 4.0

095 galbanum oil (Ferula galbaniflua) Umbelliferae (pg70)   4.0
096 galbanum resin (Ferula galbaniflua) Umbelliferae (pg107)   5.0

097 gardenia oil (Gardenia jasminoides) Rubiaceae (pg120)   not important

098 genet absolute (Spartium junceum) Leguminosae (pg100)   0.3

099 geranium oil, Algerian (Pelargonium graveolens) Geraniaceae (pg74) 10.0
100 geranium oil, Bourbon (Pelargonium graveolens) Geraniaceae (pg74) 10.0

101 geranium oil, Moroccan (Pelargonium graveolens) Geraniaceae (pg74) 10.0

102 ginger oil (Zingiber officinale) Zingiberaceae (pg69)   4.0

103 goldenrod oil (Solidago odora) Compositae (pg132)   uncertain

104 grapefruit oil, expressed (Citrus paradisi) Rutaceae (pg75)   10.0

105 guaiacwood oil (Bulnesia sarmienti) Zygophyllaceae (pg65)   8.0

106 gurjun balsam (Dipterocarpus turbinatus) Dipterocarpaceae (pg107)   5.0
107 gurjun oil (Dipterocarpus turbinatus) Dipterocarpaceae (pg66)   8.0

108 heterotheca oil (Heterotheca latifolia) Compositae (pg133)   uncertain

109 hibawood oil (Thujopsis dolabrata) Cupressaceae (pg62)   10.0

110 hinoki oil (Chamaecyparis obtusa) Cupressaceae (pg127)   (tentative) 10.0

111 ho leaf oil (Cinnamomum camphora) Lauraceae (pg78)   10.0

112 honeysuckle absolute (Lonicera caprifolium) Caprifoliaceae (pg101)   3.0

113 horseradish oil (Amoracia rusticana) Cruciferae (pg116)   **do not use**

114 hyacinth absolute (Hyacinthus orientalis) Liliaceae (pg102)   8.0

115 hyssop oil (Hyssopus officinalis) Labiatae (pg82)   4.0

116 immortelle absolute (Helichrysum angustifolium) Compositae (pg99) 2.0
117 immortelle oil (Helichrysum angustifolium) Compositae (pg67)   4.0

118 jasmine absolute (Jasminum officinale) Oleaceae (pg98)   3.0

119 jonquil absolute (Narcissus jonquilla) Amaryllidaceae (pg103)   2.0

120 juniper berry oil (Juniperus communis) Cupressaceae (pg65)   8.0
121 juniper oil, Phoenician (Juniperus phoenicia) Cupressaceae (pg73)   1.0

122 karo karounde absolute (Leptactina senegambica) Rubiaceae (pg102) 1.0

123 kesom oil (Polygonum minus) Polygonaceae (pg128)   uncertain

124 labdanum/cyste absolute (Cistus ladaniferus) Cistaceae (pg99)   3.0
125 labdanum/cyste oil (Cistus ladaniferus) Cistaceae (pg64)   8.0

126 laurel leaf oil (Laurus nobilis) Lauraceae (pg77)   2.0

127 lavandin absolute (Lavandula hybrida) Labiatae (pg99)   3.0
128 lavandin oil (Lavandula hybrida) Labiatae (pg71)   4.0
129 lavender absolute (Lavandula officinalis) Labiatae (pg99)   3.0
130 lavender oil (Lavandula officinalis) Labiatae (pg62)   15.0
131 lavender oil, spike/aspic (Lavandula latifolia) Labiatae (pg74)   8.0

132 layana oil (Artemisia afra) Compositae (pg128)   2.0

133 lemon oil, distilled (Citrus limon) Rutaceae (pg64)   10.0
134 lemon oil, expressed (Citrus limon) Rutaceae (pg75)   8.0

135 lemongrass oil, E. Indian (Cymbopogon citratus) Graminae (pg69)   4.0
136 lemongrass oil, W. Indian (Cymbopogon citratus) Graminae (pg69)   4.0

137 lemonmint oil (Mentha citrata) Labiatae (pg64)	8.0
138 licorice oil (Glycyrrhiza glabra) Leguminosae (pg122)	uncertain
139 lilac oil (Syringa vulgaris) Oleaceae (pg119)	not important
140 lily-of-the-valley oil (Convallaria majalis) Liliaceae (pg119)	not important
141 lime oil, distilled (Citrus aurantifolia) Rutaceae (pg61)	15.0
142 lime oil, expressed (Citrus aurantifolia) Rutaceae (pg75)	4.0
143 linaloe wood oil (Bursera delpechiana) Burseraceae (pg65)	8.0
144 litsea oil (Litsea cubeba) Lauraceae (pg66)	8.0
145 lovage oil (Levisticum officinale) Umbelliferae (pg78)	2.0
146 mace oil (Myristica fragans) Myristicaceae (pg77)	8.0
147 magnolia oil (Magnolia grandiflora) Magnoliaceae (pg126)	not important
148 mandarin oil, expressed (Citrus nobilis) Rutaceae (pg75)	10.0
149 marjoram oil (Origanum marjorana) Labiatae (pg80)	4.0
150 massoia oil (Cryptocaria massoia) Lauraceae (pg128)	uncertain
151 mastic absolute (Pistacia lentiscus) Anacardiaceae (pg103)	3.0

152 melissa oil (Melissa officinalis) Labiatae (pg112)	uncertain
153 mignonette oil (Reseda odorata) Resedaceae (pg120)	not important
154 mimosa absolute (Acacia decurrens) Leguminosae (pg103)	1.0
155 monarda oil (Monarda fistulosa) Labiatae (pg133)	uncertain
156 muhuhu oil (Brachylaena hutchinsii) Compositae (pg130)	uncertain
157 mustard oil (Brassica nigra) Cruciferae (pg116)	**do not use**
158 myrrh absolute (Commiphora myrrha) Burseraceae (pg104)	3.0
159 myrrh oil (Commiphora myrrha) Burseraceae (pg81)	8.0
160 myrtle oil (Myrtus communis) Myrtaceae (pg67)	4.0
161 narcissus absolute (Narcissus poetieus) Amaryllidaceae (pg103)	2.0
162 neroli/orange flower absolute (Citrus aurantium) Rutaceae (pg98)	3.0
163 neroli/orange flower oil (Citrus aurantium) Rutaceae (pg70)	4.0
164 nutmeg oil (Myristica fragans) Myristicaceae (pg79)	2.0
165 oakmoss concrete (Evernia prunastri) Usneaceae (pg106)	**do not use**
166 olibanum absolute (Boswellia carterii) Burseraceae (pg99)	3.0
167 olibanum gum (Boswellia carterii) Burseraceae (pg107)	5.0
168 olibanum oil (Boswellia carterii) Burseraceae (pg123)	(tentative) 8.0

169 opoponax absolute (Opoponax chironium) Umbelliferae (pg115)	8.0
170 bitter orange oil, expressed (Citrus aurantium) Rutaceae (pg75)	8.0
171 sweet orange oil, expressed (Citrus sinensis) Rutaceae (pg75)	10.0
172 oregano oil (Origanum vulgare) Labiatae (pg92)	0.5
173 orris absolute (Iris pallida) Iridaceae (pg100)	3.0
174 osmanthus oil (Osmanthus fragrans) Oleaceae (pg127)	uncertain
175 palmarosa oil (Cymbopogon martini) Graminae (pg55)	8.0
176 parsley herb oil (Petroselinum sativum) Umbelliferae (pg78)	2.0
177 parsley seed oil (Petroselinum sativum) Umbelliferae (pg76)	2.0
178 parsnip root oil (Pastinaca sativa) Umbelliferae (pg115)	uncertain
179 patchouli oil (Pogostemon cablin) Labiatae (pg63)	10.0
180 pennyroyal oil (Mentha pulegium) Labiatae (pg85)	2.0
181 pepper oil, black (Piper nigrum) Piperaceae (pg69)	4.0
182 peppermint oil (Mentha piperita) Labiatae (pg112)	(tentative) 4.0
183 perilla oil (Perilla frutescens) Labiatae (pg87)	0.5

184 Peru balsam (Myroxylon pereirae) Leguminosae (pg108)	do not use
185 Peru balsam oil (Myroxylon pereirae) Leguminosae (pg80)	8.0
186 Peruvian mastic oil (Schinus molle) Anacardiaceae (pg68)	4.0
187 petitgrain oil, Bigarade (Citrus aurantium) Rutaceae (pg65)	8.0
188 petitgrain oil, Paraguay (Citrus aurantium) Rutaceae (pg65)	8.0
189 petitgrain oil, lemon (Citrus limon) Rutaceae (pg64)	10.0
190 pimento berry oil (Pimenta officinalis) Myrtaceae (pg91)	4.0
191 pimento leaf oil (Pimenta officinalis) Myrtaceae (pg91)	4.0
192 pine oil, pumilo (Pinus pumilo) Pinaceae (pg86)	1.0
193 pine oil, yarmor (Pinus palustris) Pinaceae (pg78)	4.0
194 pine oil, Scots (Pinus sylvestris) Pinaceae (pg62)	10.0
195 pteronia oil (Pteronia incana) Compositae (pg129)	uncertain
196 rose absolute, French (Rosa centifolia) Rosaceae (pg98)	2.0
197 rose oil, Bulgarian (Rosa damascena) Rosaceae (pg74)	2.0
198 rose oil, Moroccan (Rosa centifolia) Rosaceae (pg74)	2.0
199 rose oil, Turkish (Rosa damascena) Rosaceae (pg74)	2.0
200 rosemary oil (Rosmarinus officinalis) Labiatae (pg63)	10.0
201 rue oil (Ruta graveolens) Rutaceae (pg88)	0.5
202 sage oil, clary French (Salvia sclarea) Labiatae (pg74)	8.0
203 sage oil, clary Russian (Salvia sclarea) Labiatae (pg74)	8.0
204 sage oil, Dalmatian (Salvia officinalis) Labiatae (pg79)	8.0
205 sage oil, Spanish (Salvia lavandulaefolia) Labiatae (pg64)	8.0

206 sandalwood oil (Santalum album) Santalaceae (pg63)	10.0
207 santolina oil (Santolina chamaecyparissus) Compositae (pg114) (tentative)	2.0
208 sassafras oil (Sassafras albidum) Lauraceae (pg94)	**do not use**
209 savin oil (Juniperus sabina) Cupressaceae (pg118)	**do not use**
210 savory oil, summer (Satureja hortensis) Labiatae (pg92)	0.5
211 skimmia oil (Skimmia laureola) Lauraceae (pg125)	uncertain
212 snakeroot oil (Asarum canadense) Aristolochiaceae (pg70)	4.0
213 Spanish marjoram oil (Thymus mastichina) Labiatae (pg71)	4.0
214 Spanish oregano oil (Thymus capitatus) Labiatae (pg113)	(tentative) 8.0
215 spearmint oil (Mentha spicata) Labiatae (pg70)	4.0
216 spikenard oil (Nardostachys jatamansi) Valerianaceae (pg124) (tentative)	10.0
217 spruce oil (Picea mariana & glauca) Pinaceae (pg73)	1.0
218 star anise oil (Illicium verum) Illiciaceae (pg79)	4.0
219 storax resinoid (Styrax officinalis) Styracaceae (pg115)	4.0
220 tagetes oil (Tagetes minuta) Compositae (pg87)	0.25

221 tangerine oil, expressed (Citrus reticulata) Rutaceae (pg75)		10.0
222 tangelo oil, expressed (Citrus reticulata x paradisi) Rutaceae (pg75)		8.0
223 tansy oil (Tanacetum vulgare) Compositae (pg83)		4.0
224 tarragon oil (Artemisia dracunculus) Compositae (pg80)		4.0
225 tea tree oil (Melaleuca alternifolia) Myrtaceae (pg81)		1.0
226 tejpat oil (Cinnamomum tamala) Lauraceae (pg124)	(tentative)	10.0
227 Texas cedarwood oil (Juniperus mexicana) Cupressaceae (pg86)		1.0
228 thuja leaf oil (Thuja occidentalis) Cupressaceae (pg84)		2.0
229 thyme oil, garden red (Thymus vulgaris) Labiatae (pg64)	(tentative)	8.0
230 thyme oil, wild (Thymus serphyllum) Labiatae (pg113)		8.0
231 tobacco leaf absolute (Nicotiana affinis) Solanaceae (pg101)		1.0
232 Tolu balsam (Myroxylon balsamum) Leguminosae (pg108)		2.0
233 tonka absolute (Dipteryx odorata) Leguminosae (pg102)		3.0
234 treemoss concrete (Usnea barbata) Usneaceae (pg106)		**do not use**
235 tuberose absolute (Polianthus tuberosa) Agavaceae (pg133)		not important

236 turmeric oil (Curcuma longa) Zingiberaceae (pg69)	4.0
237 valerian oil (Valeriana officinalis) Valerianaceae (pg115)	uncertain
238 vanilla tincture (Vanilla planifolia) Orchidaceae (pg104)	3.0
239 vassoura oil (Baccharis dracunculifolia) Compositae (pg132)	uncertain
240 vateria oil (Vateria indica) Dipterocarpaceae (pg124)	uncertain
241 verbena absolute (Lippia citriodora) Verbenaceae (pg103)	**do not use**
242 verbena oil (Lippia citriodora) Verbenaceae (pg89)	0.25
243 vetivert oil (Vetiveria zizanoides) Graminae (pg65)	8.0
244 violet leaf absolute (Viola odorata) Violaceae (pg99)	2.0
245 Virginian cedarwood oil (Juniperus virginiana) Cupressaceae (pg86)	1.0
246 wintergreen oil (Gaultheria procumbens) Ericaceae (pg117-8)	**do not use**
247 wormwood oil (Artemisia absinthium) Compositae (pg83)	2.0
248 yarrow oil (Achillea millefolium) Compositae (pg113)	(tentative) 4.0
249 ylang-ylang oil (Cananga odorata) Annonaceae (pg63)	10.0
250 zdravetz oil (Geranium macrorrhizum) Geraniaceae (pg114)	uncertain

References for the Monographs

The original RIFM monographs were published in the 'Food and Cosmetic Toxicology' journal* by Pergamon Press, United Kingdom. Monographs used in this guide are selected from the 1973 to 1992 issues. References for the information found in this guide are too numerous to include. They can be found in the original monographs, the locations of which are listed below in chronological order as they appeared in the journal. The numbers of pages are given in brackets.

* The name of this journal has been changed from Vol.20 (1982) onwards to 'Food and Chemical Toxicology'.

Vol.11 No.5 (Oct 1973)
amyris oil [acetylated]   pgs.861 (1)
anise oil   pgs.865-866 (2)
basil oil, sweet   pgs.897-868 (2)
bay oil   pgs.869-870 (2)
benzoin resinoid   pgs.871-872 (2)

Vol.11 No.6 (Dec 1973)
bergamot oil, expressed   pgs.1031-1033 (3)
bergamot oil, rectified   pgs.1035 (1)
birch tar oil   pgs.1037 (1)
bois de rose oil [acetylated] pgs.1039 (1)
camphor oil, white   pgs.1047 (1)
cananga oil   pgs.1049 (1)
caraway oil   pgs.1051 (1)
citronella oil   pgs.1067-1068 (2)
copaiba oil   pgs.1075 (1)
coriander oil   pgs.1077 (1)

Vol.12 No.3 (Jun 1974)
cyste absolute   pgs.403 (1)

Vol.12 No.5/6 (Oct 1974)
estragon (tarragon) oil   pgs.709 (1)
grapefruit oil, expressed   pgs.723-724 (2)
lemon oil, expressed   pgs.725-726 (2)
lemon oil, distilled   pgs.727 (1)
lime oil, distilled   pgs.729 (1)
lime oil, expressed   pgs.731 (1)
(sweet) orange oil, expressed pgs.733-734 (2)
bitter orange oil, expressed   pgs.735-736 (2)

Vol.12 Supplement - Special Issue I (Dec 1974) - *foreword by Leon Goldberg.*

Abies alba (silver fir cone) oil	pgs.809-810 (2)
Abies alba (silver fir needle) oil	pgs.811 (1)
angelica seed oil	pgs.821 (1)
cardamom oil	pgs.837-838 (2)
cedarleaf oil	pgs.843-844 (2)
Virginian cedarwood oil	pgs.845-846 (2)
celery seed oil	pgs.849-850 (2)
chamomile oil, German	pgs.851-852 (2)
chamomile oil, Roman	pgs.853 (1)
clary sage oil (French)	pgs.865-866 (2)
costus root oil, absolute & concrete	pgs.867-868 (2)
cumin oil	pgs.869-870 (2)
fennel oil (sweet)	pgs.879-880 (2)
geranium oil, Bourbon	pgs.883-884 (2)
ginger oil	pgs.901-902 (2)
guaiac wood oil	pgs.905 (1)
ho leaf oil	pgs.917 (1)
oregano oil	pgs.945-946 (2)
palmarosa oil	pgs.947 (1)
pennyroyal oil, Eurafrican	pgs.949-950 (2)
peru balsam	pgs.951-952 (2)
peru balsam oil	pgs.953-954 (2)
pimento leaf oil	pgs.971-972 (2)
rosemary oil	pgs.977-978 (2)
rose oil, Bulgarian	pgs.979-980 (2)
rose oil, Moroccan	pgs.981-982 (2)
sage oil, Dalmatian	pgs.987-988 (2)
sandalwood oil, East Indian	pgs.989-990 (2)
thyme oil, red	pgs.1003-1004 (2)
tonka absolute	pgs.1005 (1)
vetiver oil	pgs.1013 (1)
ylang-ylang oil	pgs.1015-1016 (2)

Vol.13 No.1 (Feb 1975)

eucalyptus oil	pgs.107-108 (2)
cassia oil	pgs.109-110 (2)
cinnamon bark oil, Ceylon	pgs.111-112 (2)

Vol.13 No.4 (Aug 1975) [mixed-up - monographs not given a fresh page each as per usual !]

(fir) balsam, Canadian	pgs.449 (1)
fir needle oil, Canadian	pgs.450 (1)
fir needle oil, Siberian	pgs.451 (1)
geranium oil, Moroccan	pgs.452 (1)
rue oil	pgs.456 (1)

Vol.13 Supplement - Special Issue II (Dec 1975) - *foreword by R. R. Suskind.*

ambrette seed oil	pgs.705 (1)
angelica root oil	pgs.713-714 (2)
star anise oil	pgs.715-716 (2)
armoise oil	pgs.719 (1)
wormwood oil	pgs.721-722 (2)
cade (tar) oil, rectified	pgs.733-734 (2)
camphor oil, yellow	pgs.739-740 (2)
cinnamon leaf oil, Ceylon	pgs.749 (1)
clove bud oil	pgs.761-763 (3)
clove stem oil	pgs.765-767 (3)
cognac oil, green	pgs.769 (1)
cornmint oil	pgs.771-772 (2)
mimosa absolute	pgs.873-874 (2)
oakmoss concrete	pgs.891-892 (2)
orris absolute	pgs.895-895 (2)
parsley seed oil	pgs.897-898 (2)
rose absolute, French	pgs.911-912 (2)
rose oil, Turkish	pgs.913 (1)
treemoss concrete	pgs.915-917 (3)

Vol.14 No.4 (Aug 1976)

alantroot (elecampane) oil	pgs.307-308 (2)
fennel oil, bitter	pgs.309 (1)* - refer to Vol.17 No.5 (Oct 1979)
jasmine absolute	pgs.331 (1)
juniper berry oil	pgs.333 (1)
labdanum oil	pgs.335 (1)
laurel leaf oil	pgs.337-338 (2)

Vol.14 No.5 (Oct 1976)

lavandin oil [acetylated]	pgs.445 (1)
lavandin oil	pgs.447 (1)
lavender absolute	pgs.449 (1)
lavender oil	pgs.451 (1)
lavender oil, spike	pgs.453 (1)
lemongrass oil, East Indian	pgs.455 (1)
lemongrass oil, West Indian	pgs.457 (1)
Spanish marjoram oil	pgs.467 (1)
marjoram oil, sweet	pgs.469 (1)

Vol.14 No.6 (Dec 1976)
myrrh oil   pgs.621 (1)
nutmeg oil, East Indian   pgs.631-633 (3)

Vol.14 Supplement - Special Issue III (Dec 1976) - *foreword by Howard Spencer.*
copaiba balsam   pgs.687 (1)
tolu balsam   pgs.689-690 (2)
cajeput oil   pgs.701 (1)
camphor oil, brown   pgs.703 (1)
carrot seed oil   pgs.705-706 (2)
cascarilla oil   pgs.707 (1)
cedarwood oil, Atlas   pgs.709 (1)
Texas cedarwood oil   pgs.711-712 (2)
chenopodium oil   pgs.713-715 (3)
cubeb oil   pgs.729-730 (2)
davana oil   pgs.737 (1)
dill weed/herb oil   pgs.747-748 (2)
eau de brouts absolute   pgs.753 (1)
elemi oil   pgs.755 (1)
foin absolute   pgs.777 (1)
genet absolute   pgs.779 (1)
geranium oil, Algerian   pgs.781-782 (2)
gurjun balsam   pgs.789-790 (2)
gurjun oil   pgs.791 (1)
hyacinth absolute   pgs.795 (1)
neroli (orange flower) oil, Tunisian   pgs.813-814 (2)
Pinus pumilo oil   pgs.843-844 (2)
Pinus slyvestris oil   pgs.845-846 (2)
sage oil, Spanish   pgs.857-858 (2)
savory oil, summer   pgs.859-860 (2)
(Peruvian mastic) Schinus molle oil   pgs.861 (1)
tansy oil   pgs.869-871 (3)
violet leaf absolute   pgs.893 (1)

Vol.15 No.6 (Dec 1977)
calamus oil   pgs.623-626 (4)

Vol.16 Supplement - Special Issue IV (Dec 1978) - *foreword by K. E. Malten.*
black pepper oil	pgs.651-652 (2)
bois de rose oil, Brazilian	pgs.653-654 (2)
clove leaf oil, Madagascar	pgs.695 (1)
cypress oil	pgs.699 (1)
fenugreek absolute	pgs.755-756 (2)
flouve oil	pgs.757 (1)
galbanum oil	pgs.765-766 (2)
(immortelle) helichrysum oil	pgs.769-770 (2)
hyssop oil	pgs.783-784 (2)
petitgrain oil, lemon	pgs.807 (1)
lovage oil	pgs.813-814 (2)
narcissus absolute	pgs.827 (1)
(Brazilian sassafras) Ocotea cymbarum oil	pgs.831 (1)
olibanum absolute	pgs.835 (1)
olibanum gum	pgs.837 (1)
snakeroot oil, Canadian	pgs.869-870 (2)
spearmint oil	pgs.871-872 (2)
tangerine oil, expressed	pgs.873-874 (2)
tobacco leaf absolute	pgs.875 (1)

Vol.17 No.4 (Aug 1979)
(Douglas) fir balsam, Oregon	pgs.369-370 (2)
pimento berry oil	pgs.381 (1)

Vol.17 No.5 (Oct 1979)
fennel oil, bitter	pgs.529 (1)*

[The results in the monograph on fennel oil, bitter of Vol.14 No.4 pg.309 August 1976 were found to be determined from test samples that had deteriorated because of atmospheric oxidation causing an increase in the levels of p-cymene above 2% and anisic aldehyde above 0.3%. The results in this monograph were obtained from tests using a fresh sample.]

Vol.17 Supplement - Special Issue V (Dec 1979) - *foreword by Donald Birmingham M.D.*
ale oil	pgs.701 (1)
almond oil, bitter	pgs.705-706 (2)
almond oil, bitter [FFPA]	pgs.707 (1)
hibawood oil	pgs.817 (1)
immortelle absolute	pgs.821 (1)
linaloe wood oil	pgs.849 (1)
mace oil	pgs.851-852 (2)
sweet birch oil	pgs.907 (1)

Vol.20 Supplement - Special Issue VI (Nov 1982) - *foreword by Masaru Ishihara.*

boldo leaf oil	pgs.643-644 (2)
carbreuva oil	pgs.645 (1)
dill seed oil, Indian	pgs.673-674 (2)
fig leaf absolute	pgs.691-692 (2)
Litsea cubeba oil	pgs.731-732 (2)
(neroli) orange flower absolute	pgs.785 (1)
patchouly oil	pgs.791-793 (3)
petitgrain oil, Paraguay	pgs.801-802 (2)
sage clary oil, Russian	pgs.823-824 (2)
sassafras oil	pgs.825-826 (2)
tagetes oil	pgs.829-830 (2)
tangelo oil (expressed)	pgs.831 (1)
vanilla tincture	pgs.849-850 (2)

Vol.21 No. 6 (Dec 1983)

(turmeric) curcuma oil	pgs.839-841 (3)
jonquil absolute	pgs.861 (1)
yarmor pine oil	pgs.875 (1)
myrtle oil	pgs.869-870 (2)
parsley herb oil	pgs.871-872 (2)

Vol.26 Supplement - Special Issue VII (1988) - *foreword by R. A. Ford.*

Eucalyptus citridora oil	pgs.323 (1)
honeysuckle absolute	pgs.357 (1)
perilla oil	pgs.397-8 (2)
tea tree oil	pgs.407 (1)

Vol.30 Supplement - Special Issue VIII (1992) - *foreword by Thomas Lawley.*

Eucalyptus citriodora oil [acetylated]	pgs.35 (1)
galbanum resin	pgs.39 (1)
Juniperus phoenicia oil	pgs.59 (1)
karo karonde absolute	pgs.61 (1)
lavandin absolute	pgs.65 (1)
mandarin oil, expressed	pgs.69-90 (2)
mastic absolute	pgs.71-2 (2)
(lemonmint) Mentha citrata oil	pgs.73 (1)
myrrh absolute	pgs.91 (1)
petitgrain, Bigarade oil	pgs.101 (1)
spruce oil	pgs.117-8 (2)
verbena absolute	pgs.135 (1)
verbena oil	pgs.137-8 (2)

Endnote

The RIFM also published a monograph on sweet almond oil which is a fixed oil and not an essential oil. It is therefore not included in the listing of fragrance materials in this book. Sweet almond oil has a moderate rate of absorption and is used extensively up to 30ml at a time in aromatherapy as a carrier for the essential oils, without any adverse effects. It is mentioned here for completeness.

The original RIFM monograph on sweet almond oil was published in the 'Food and Cosmetic Toxicology' journal Vol. 17 Supplement - Special Issue V pg. 709 (Dec 1979).

Five additional monographs were published by the RIFM on natural fragrance materials from animal origin. Since aromatherapy uses natural plant extracts exclusively, these animal fragrance materials are excluded from this book.

Anyone interested in them will find safety information in the same journal for the following:

ambergris (tincture) - alcohol extraction of the gastric or intestinal secretion of the sperm whale (Physeter catadon). Vol.14 Special Issue III pgs.675 (1976)

musk (tincture) - alcohol extraction of the glandular secretion of the male musk deer (Moschus moschiferus). Vol.12 No.6 pgs.865 (1983)

civet (absolute) - alcohol extraction of the glandular secretion of both sexes of the civet (Viverra civetta). Vol.12 Special Issue I pgs.863 (1974)

castoreum (tincture) - alcohol extraction of the secretion from the oil glands of the beaver (Castor fiber). Vol.11 No.6 pgs.1061 (1973)

beeswax (absolute) - alcohol extraction of the raw wax from the honeycomb of the bee (Apis mellifera). Vol.14 Special Issue III pgs.691 (1976)

The **International School of Aromatherapy (ISA)** is one of the institutions in the United Kingdom actively involved in the professional training of aromatherapists. To support its educational programme, the ISA maintains a reference library with a computer database of several thousand bibliographic references of scientific research on all aspects of essential oils. The references were abstracted from the world's foremost medical and biological science databases including **Index Medicus**, **Excerpta Medica**, **FSTA**, **Biosis** and **Science Citation Index**. A printed copy of all the important articles is also filed in the library to provide a single comprehensive source of information in this field for aromatherapy students. This facility has been used by visiting students from several universities researching for their papers.

'A Safety Guide on the use of Essential Oils' @ £12.00 is available from:

Natural by Nature Oils Ltd.
9 Vivian Avenue
Hendon Central
LONDON NW4 3UT

The Natural by Nature Oils company is a commercial supplier of fine quality essential oils for exclusive use in aromatherapy. This company is concerned with public safety in the use of essential oils and financed the compilation and publication of this safety guide book as a consumer information service.

As more information becomes available from further research,
the contents of this book will be updated.

The staff of the International School of Aromatherapy is unable to reply to
enquiries personally. However readers' suggestions and comments are welcomed
and will be considered in the revision of further editions.

**Please direct all letters to the Course Director,
International School of Aromatherapy,
c/o the publisher's address as above.**